Nutritionist's Ninja Creami Recipes For Beginners 2025

Healthy Guilt-Free Treats with Nutritious Ingredients

Clara Winslow, CN

DISCLAIMER

The information, including but not limited to, text, graphics, images and other material contained in this guide are for informational purposes only. No material from this guide is intended to be a substitute for professional medical advice, diagnosis or treatment.

Always seek the advice of your physician or other qualified health care provider with any questions you may have regarding a medical condition or treatment and before undertaking a new health care regimen, and never disregard professional medical advice or delay in seeking it because of something you have read in this guide.

Table of CONTENTS

INTRODUCTION

Welcome to the Ninja Creami Cookbook

Welcome to **The Nutritionist's Ninja Creami Healthy Recipes Cookbook 2025: Healthy Guilt-Free Treats with Nutritious Ingredients**! I'm thrilled to have you join me on this delicious journey to create a variety of wholesome frozen treats that cater to your health-conscious lifestyle. This cookbook is designed with you in mind—whether you are a busy professional, a dedicated parent, or simply someone who loves to indulge in sweet delights without the guilt, you'll find an array of nutritious recipes that are easy to prepare and absolutely delightful to enjoy.

Homemade frozen treats allow you to take control of your ingredients, ensuring that you can enjoy desserts made with wholesome, natural components while avoiding artificial additives and excessive sugars. With the versatile Ninja Creami, you'll be able to whip up everything from creamy ice creams to refreshing sorbets in a matter of minutes. Each recipe is crafted to be both satisfying and nutritious, helping you to meet your health goals while enjoying the flavors you love.

Clara Winslow's **Story**

I'm Clara Winslow, a certified nutritionist with a passion for healthy cooking and family nutrition. Growing up in a household that cherished homemade treats, I developed a deep appreciation for the flavors and experiences that come from cooking together. After earning my Bachelor's degree in Nutritional Science, I embarked on a journey to empower families to embrace healthier eating habits without sacrificing the joy of delicious food.

My experience working in various healthcare settings has shown me the importance of balanced nutrition and how it can positively impact overall health. I created this cookbook to share my love for healthy desserts and to provide you with the tools and knowledge to create indulgent yet nutritious frozen treats that you can feel good about. My goal is to make healthy eating fun and accessible for everyone, proving that you can enjoy your favorite flavors while nourishing your body.

HOW TO BEST USE THIS *Cookbook*

This cookbook is structured to be user-friendly and accessible for cooks of all skill levels. You'll find a variety of recipes categorized by type, including ice creams, sorbets, smoothie bowls, and more. Each recipe includes a list of ingredients, step-by-step instructions, and a detailed nutritional breakdown, allowing you to make informed choices about what you're consuming.

As you explore the recipes, don't hesitate to get creative! The Ninja Creami allows for endless customization, so feel free to experiment with flavors, ingredients, and mix-ins to suit your family's preferences. You'll also find tips for ingredient substitutions and meal prep ideas throughout the book, helping you to maintain a healthy lifestyle even on your busiest days.

With the **Ninja Creami** at your side and this cookbook in hand, you're ready to embark on a flavorful journey filled with nutritious, delicious frozen treats that will bring joy to your kitchen and smiles to your family's faces. Let's get started on creating wholesome indulgences that everyone will love!

Understanding THE NINJA CREAMI

What is the *Ninja Creami?*

The **Ninja Creami** is an innovative appliance designed to simplify the process of making homemade frozen treats, such as ice creams, sorbets, and smoothie bowls. This powerful machine takes your frozen bases and transforms them into creamy, delicious desserts with minimal effort. With its user-friendly design and advanced technology, the Ninja Creami allows you to create a variety of frozen delights tailored to your dietary preferences and health goals. It's an essential tool for anyone looking to enjoy indulgent treats while maintaining a focus on nutrition.

Benefits of Using the Ninja Creami for Healthy Treats

When it comes to incorporating healthy ingredients into your desserts, the Ninja Creami shines. Here are some key benefits of using this appliance for creating nutritious frozen treats:

1. **Customizable Recipes:** The Ninja Creami allows you to experiment with different ingredients, enabling you to create recipes that cater to your dietary needs—whether you're looking for low-sugar, dairy-free, or high-protein options.
2. **Nutrient Retention:** By making your own frozen treats, you can retain the nutritional value of your ingredients. This means you can enjoy the health benefits associated with fruits, nuts, and wholesome dairy or dairy alternatives without the additives commonly found in store-bought products.
3. **Convenience and Speed:** The Ninja Creami processes your frozen bases quickly and efficiently, allowing you to whip up delicious treats in just minutes. This convenience makes it easier to fit healthy desserts into your busy lifestyle.
4. **Versatility:** This appliance is designed to handle a wide range of recipes, from creamy ice creams to refreshing sorbets and smoothie bowls. You can create a variety of flavors and textures to keep your dessert options exciting.
5. **Family-Friendly:** The Ninja Creami makes it fun to involve your family in the kitchen. Kids can help choose flavors, mix ingredients, and enjoy the end results, making healthy eating a shared experience.

Getting Started

Key Features and Functions

To make the most of your Ninja Creami, it's important to familiarize yourself with its key features and functions:

1. **Processing Functions:** The Ninja Creami offers several processing options tailored for different types of frozen treats:
   - **Ice Cream Function:** Ideal for creating rich, creamy ice creams.
   - **Sorbet Function:** Perfect for making smooth and refreshing sorbets from fruits and juices.
   - **Gelato Function:** Designed for denser, creamier results akin to traditional gelato.
   - **Mix-In Function:** Allows you to add mix-ins like chocolate chips or fruit pieces without over-processing, ensuring a delightful crunch in every bite.
2. **User-Friendly Control Panel:** The intuitive control panel features easy-to-use buttons for each processing function, along with a digital display that guides you through the process. This makes it simple for anyone to operate, regardless of cooking experience.
3. **Compact Design:** The Ninja Creami's sleek and compact design ensures it fits easily on your countertop without taking up too much space. Its stylish appearance makes it a welcome addition to any kitchen.
4. **Easy Cleanup:** All removable parts, including the pint containers and lids, are dishwasher safe, making cleanup quick and convenient. The base of the machine can be wiped down with a damp cloth, ensuring it stays tidy and ready for your next culinary creation.

By understanding the Ninja Creami's features and functions, you'll be well-equipped to create a variety of healthy frozen treats that delight your taste buds and support your nutritional goals. Let's dive into the exciting recipes that will help you unleash your creativity in the kitchen while maintaining a focus on health!

HEALTHY INGREDIENTS

for Guilt-Free Treats

Essential Ingredients for Nutritious Frozen Desserts

Base Ingredients

- **Dairy or Dairy Alternatives:** Heavy cream, Greek yogurt, and coconut cream provide a rich base for ice creams and sorbets. For dairy-free options, unsweetened almond milk, oat milk, or coconut milk offer excellent alternatives with varying flavors and textures.
- **Sweeteners:** Natural sweeteners such as honey, maple syrup, or coconut sugar can enhance the flavor of your desserts. For lower-sugar options, consider using sugar-free alternatives like erythritol, stevia, or monk fruit.
- **Fruits:** Fresh or frozen fruits are essential for adding natural sweetness and flavor. Berries, bananas, mangoes, and peaches are all excellent choices for smoothies, sorbets, and ice creams.

Protein Sources

- **Protein Powder:** Adding protein powder (whey, casein, or plant-based) to your recipes boosts the protein content, making them more satisfying and beneficial for muscle recovery.
- **Nut Butters:** Almond butter, peanut butter, or sunflower seed butter add healthy fats and protein, enhancing both flavor and texture in your frozen treats.

Texture Enhancers

- **Chia Seeds:** These tiny seeds are rich in omega-3 fatty acids and fiber. When soaked, they create a gel-like consistency that can add creaminess to smoothies and frozen desserts.
- **Gelatin or Agar-Agar:** These ingredients can be used to help thicken and stabilize ice creams and sorbets, providing a smooth texture.

Flavor Enhancers

- **Extracts and Spices:** Vanilla extract, almond extract, and spices like cinnamon and nutmeg can elevate the flavors of your desserts, making them more aromatic and enjoyable.

Tips for Choosing *Healthy Substitutes*

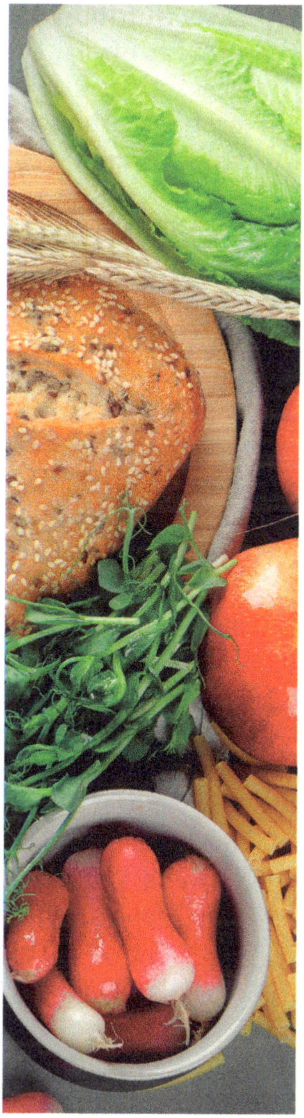

Opt for Whole Foods
Whenever possible, select whole, minimally processed ingredients. Fresh fruits, vegetables, nuts, and seeds provide essential nutrients and are generally healthier options compared to processed alternatives.

Read Labels
If you're using packaged ingredients, like protein powders or nut butters, read the labels carefully. Look for products with minimal added sugars, artificial flavors, and preservatives to ensure you're making healthful choices.

Prioritize Nutrient Density
Choose ingredients that offer a high amount of nutrients relative to their calorie content. For instance, berries provide antioxidants and vitamins while being low in calories, making them an excellent addition to your recipes.

Consider Dietary Preferences
Be mindful of dietary restrictions and preferences when selecting ingredients. Many recipes can easily be adapted to be vegan, gluten-free, or nut-free by swapping in suitable alternatives.

Nutritional Considerations for Families

Daily Nutritional Needs
Families often have varying nutritional requirements based on age, activity level, and health goals. Understanding how much protein, carbohydrates, and fats each family member needs can help you create balanced desserts.

Incorporating Variety
Ensure that your frozen treats offer a balance of flavors and nutrients. Incorporating different fruits, nuts, and seeds can provide a range of vitamins and minerals that support overall health.

Portion Control
Even healthy treats should be enjoyed in moderation. Be mindful of portion sizes, especially when it comes to high-calorie ingredients like nuts and nut butters.

Encouraging Healthy Habits
Use these recipes as a way to introduce children to the joys of cooking and healthy eating. Involving them in the preparation process can help foster a positive relationship with food and nutrition.

By focusing on these healthy ingredients and nutritional considerations, you can create guilt-free treats that nourish your family and satisfy their sweet cravings. Let's dive into the exciting recipes that will help you make the most of these wholesome ingredients while enjoying delicious frozen desserts!

FROZEN TREATS

for Every Occasion

Vanilla Almond Ice Cream

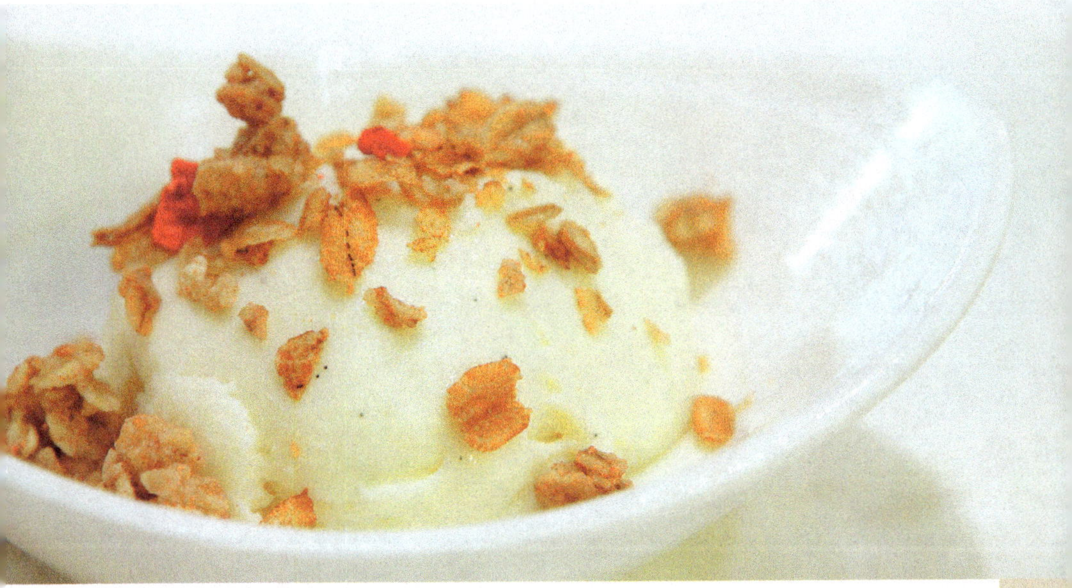

The Vanilla Almond Ice Cream is a creamy, dreamy treat that perfectly balances the classic flavor of vanilla with the nutty essence of almonds. This recipe is not only simple to prepare but also packed with wholesome ingredients, making it a fantastic choice for a healthy dessert or a delightful snack. I often whip this up for family gatherings, as it's a crowd-pleaser that appeals to both kids and adults alike. The rich almond flavor adds a unique twist to traditional vanilla ice cream, and it's a wonderful way to incorporate healthy fats and protein into your treat. Enjoy it on its own or pair it with your favorite toppings for a truly indulgent experience!

Ingredients

- 2 cups heavy cream (or coconut cream for a dairy-free option)
- 1 cup whole milk (or almond milk for a dairy-free option)
- 1/2 cup granulated sugar or your preferred sweetener (adjust to taste; can use agave syrup or erythritol for lower sugar)
- 1 tablespoon pure vanilla extract
- 1 teaspoon almond extract
- Pinch of salt
- Optional: 1/4 cup sliced almonds for added texture

Nutrition

Calories	**240**
Protein	**4 g**
Carbohydrates	**20 g**
Sugars	**10 g**
Fats (Total)	**18 g**
Saturated	**11 g**
Unsaturated	**7 g**
Fiber	**1 g**

Instructions

1. **Combine Ingredients:** In a medium saucepan, whisk together the heavy cream, whole milk, sugar (or sweetener), vanilla extract, almond extract, and a pinch of salt over medium heat until smooth and well combined.
2. **Cool the Mixture:** Allow the mixture to cool to room temperature. For quicker cooling, transfer it to a bowl and refrigerate for about 30 minutes.
3. **Freeze the Base:** Pour the cooled mixture into your Ninja Creami pint container. Ensure it's filled to the fill line and then freeze for at least 24 hours.

Creami Processing

1. **Creami Processing:** After freezing, remove the pint from the freezer. Place it in your Ninja Creami machine, select the "Ice Cream" function, and process until smooth and creamy.
2. **Add Almonds:** If you're using sliced almonds, gently fold them into the ice cream after processing for added texture.
3. **Serve or Store:** Enjoy immediately for a soft-serve texture or return to the freezer for a firmer consistency. For an extra special touch, garnish with additional sliced almonds or a drizzle of chocolate sauce before serving.

Chocolate Avocado Ice Cream

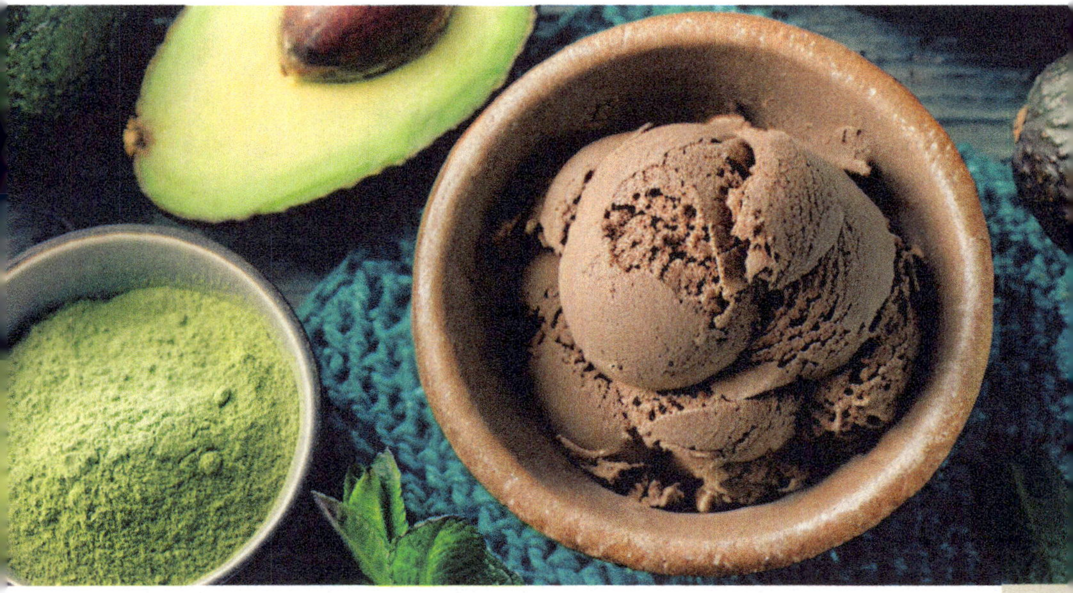

The Chocolate Avocado Ice Cream is a unique and nutritious twist on traditional chocolate ice cream. Using ripe avocados as the base adds a creamy texture and healthy fats, making this dessert both indulgent and wholesome. This recipe is perfect for anyone looking to enjoy a rich chocolate treat while benefiting from the nutritional properties of avocados. It's a favorite in my household, especially with my daughter, Emma, who loves the chocolate flavor and doesn't even realize she's getting a boost of healthy fats! This ice cream is not only delicious but also easy to make, and it's a great way to sneak in some extra nutrition.

Ingredients

- 2 ripe avocados, peeled and pitted
- 1 cup unsweetened almond milk (or any milk of choice)
- 1/2 cup unsweetened cocoa powder
- 1/2 cup maple syrup or honey (adjust to taste; can use sugar-free sweetener for lower sugar)
- 1 teaspoon pure vanilla extract
- Pinch of salt
- Optional: 1/4 cup dark chocolate chips or chunks (dairy-free if needed)

Nutrition

Calories	**220**
Protein	**4 g**
Carbohydrates	**30 g**
Sugars	**10 g**
Fats (Total)	**12 g**
Saturated	**3 g**
Unsaturated	**9 g**
Fiber	**6 g**

Instructions

1. **Blend the Ingredients:** In a blender or food processor, combine the ripe avocados, almond milk, cocoa powder, maple syrup (or honey), vanilla extract, and a pinch of salt. Blend until smooth and creamy, scraping down the sides as necessary.
2. **Taste and Adjust:** Taste the mixture and adjust sweetness if needed by adding more maple syrup or honey. Blend again if you make any adjustments to ensure everything is well combined.
3. **Chill the Mixture:** Transfer the mixture to a bowl and refrigerate for about 30 minutes to chill before freezing.
4. **Freeze the Base:** Pour the chilled mixture into your Ninja Creami pint container. Ensure it's filled to the fill line and then freeze for at least 24 hours.

Creami Processing

1. **Creami Processing:** After freezing, remove the pint from the freezer. Place it in your Ninja Creami machine, select the "Ice Cream" function, and process until smooth and creamy.
2. **Add Chocolate Chips:** If using, gently fold in the dark chocolate chips after processing for added texture and richness.
3. **Serve or Store:** Enjoy immediately for a soft-serve texture or return to the freezer for a firmer consistency. For a decorative touch, serve with a sprinkle of cocoa powder or extra chocolate chips on top.

Nutritionist Tips

- **Choosing Avocados:** Make sure to use ripe avocados for the best flavor and texture. They should be slightly soft to the touch but not overly mushy.

Strawberry Banana Sorbet

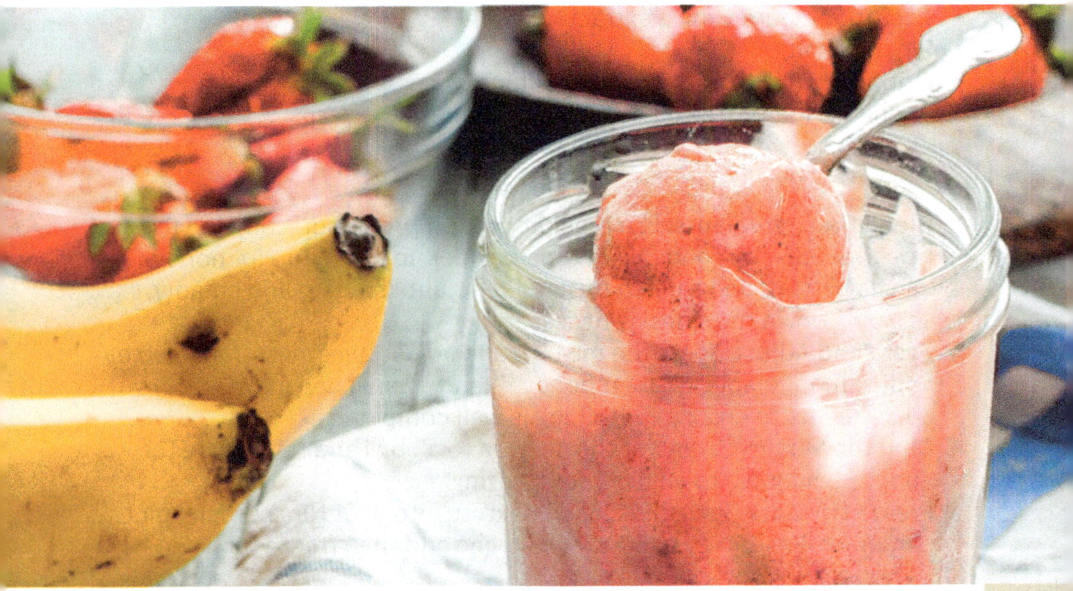

The Strawberry Banana Sorbet is a wonderfully refreshing treat that captures the delightful flavors of ripe strawberries and bananas in every scoop. This sorbet is not only incredibly easy to make but also a fantastic way to enjoy a guilt-free dessert that's naturally sweet and packed with vitamins. It's a go-to recipe in my home, especially during the warmer months when fresh strawberries are in season. I love making this sorbet with my daughter, Emma, as it's a fun way to introduce her to the joys of healthy eating while enjoying the vibrant colors and flavors of the fruits. Plus, it's dairy-free and perfect for those looking for a light, fruity dessert!

Ingredients

- 2 cups fresh strawberries, hulled and sliced (or frozen strawberries, thawed)
- 1 medium ripe banana, sliced (fresh or frozen)
- 1/2 cup unsweetened almond milk (or any milk of choice)
- 2 tablespoons honey or maple syrup (optional, adjust to taste)
- Juice of 1 lemon (about 2 tablespoons)
- Pinch of salt

Nutrition

Calories	**120**
Protein	**1 g**
Carbohydrates	**30 g**
Sugars	**18 g**
Fats (Total)	**0.5 g**
Saturated	**0 g**
Unsaturated	**0.5 g**
Fiber	**2 g**

Instructions

1. **Prepare the Fruit:** If using fresh strawberries, rinse them under cold water and hull them. If using frozen strawberries, allow them to thaw slightly for easier blending.
2. **Blend the Mixture:** In a blender, combine the strawberries, banana, almond milk, honey (if using), lemon juice, and a pinch of salt. Blend until smooth and creamy.
3. **Taste and Adjust:** Taste the mixture and adjust sweetness if necessary by adding more honey or maple syrup. Blend again if you make any adjustments.
4. **Freeze the Mixture:** Pour the blended mixture into your Ninja Creami pint container. Ensure it's filled to the fill line and then freeze for at least 24 hours.

Creami Processing

1. **Creami Processing:** After freezing, remove the pint from the freezer. Place it in your Ninja Creami machine, select the "Sorbet" function, and process until smooth.
2. **Serve or Store:** Enjoy immediately for a refreshing soft-serve texture or return to the freezer for a firmer consistency. For an extra touch, garnish with fresh strawberry slices or a sprinkle of granola before serving.

Nutritionist Tips

- **Choosing Ripe Fruits:** For the best flavor, use ripe strawberries and bananas. The natural sweetness of the fruits will enhance the overall taste of the sorbet.

Tropical Mango Smoothie Bowl

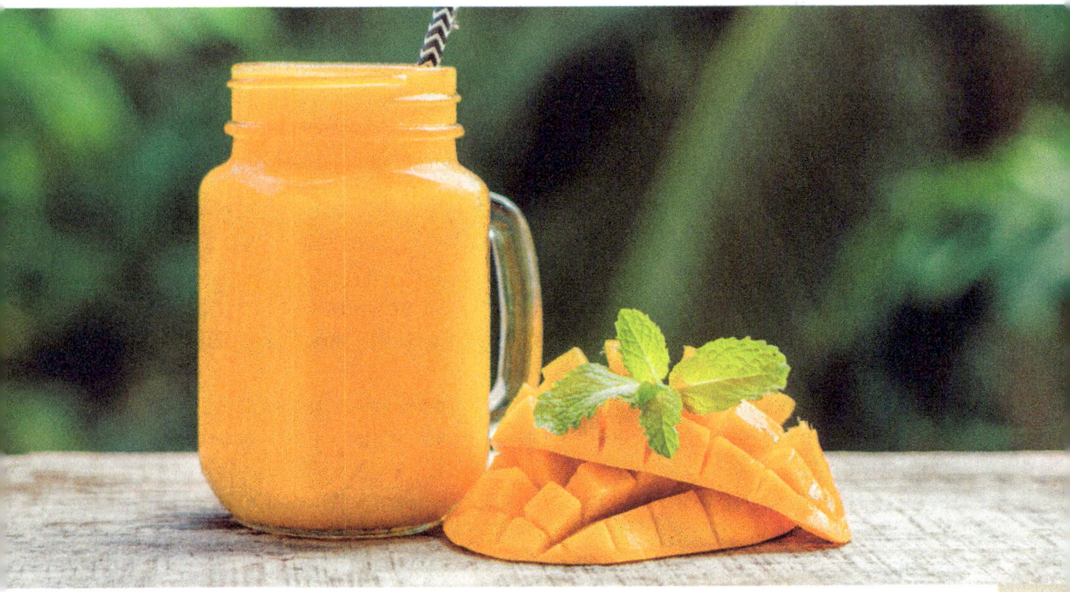

The Tropical Mango Smoothie Bowl is a vibrant, refreshing dish that brings the taste of a sunny beach right to your kitchen. Bursting with the sweet flavors of ripe mango, this smoothie bowl is not only delicious but also packed with nutrients, making it a perfect breakfast or a delightful snack. I love preparing this bowl as a fun way to start the day or to cool off after a workout. The beautiful colors and textures invite creativity, allowing you to top it with your favorite fruits, nuts, and seeds. This recipe is a hit with my family, especially Emma, who enjoys customizing her bowl with a variety of toppings!

Ingredients

- 1 ripe mango, peeled and diced (fresh or frozen)
- 1 ripe banana (fresh or frozen)
- 1/2 cup unsweetened coconut milk (or any milk of choice)
- 1/2 cup spinach or kale (optional, for added nutrients)
- 1 tablespoon chia seeds (optional, for added fiber)
- Toppings: sliced fresh fruit (such as kiwi, berries, or banana), granola, shredded coconut, and nuts or seeds

Nutrition

Calories	**250**
Protein	**4 g**
Carbohydrates	**42 g**
Sugars	**20 g**
Fats (Total)	**6 g**
Saturated	**4 g**
Unsaturated	**2 g**
Fiber	**5 g**

Instructions

1. **Blend the Base:** In a blender, combine the diced mango, banana, coconut milk, spinach or kale (if using), and chia seeds (if using). Blend until smooth and creamy.
2. **Adjust Consistency:** If the mixture is too thick, add a little more coconut milk to achieve your desired consistency. Blend again until smooth.
3. **Pour into a Bowl:** Pour the smoothie mixture into a bowl, creating a smooth, even layer.
4. **Add Toppings:** Decorate the top of your smoothie bowl with your choice of sliced fresh fruit, granola, shredded coconut, and nuts or seeds. Get creative and arrange them in a visually appealing way!
5. **Serve Immediately:** Enjoy your Tropical Mango Smoothie Bowl right away for the best flavor and texture.

Nutritionist Tips

- **Choosing Mangoes:** For the best flavor, select ripe mangoes that yield slightly to pressure when squeezed. They should be fragrant and brightly colored.
- **Frozen Fruits:** Using frozen fruits can help create a thicker, creamier texture, making it even more enjoyable.
- **Customization:** Feel free to mix in other tropical fruits such as pineapple or papaya for additional flavors and nutrients. You can also add protein powder for an extra protein boost.
- **Serving Suggestions:** This smoothie bowl can be enjoyed for breakfast, as a post-workout snack, or even as a light dessert. It's versatile and can easily fit into any meal plan!

Berry Bliss Smoothie Bowl

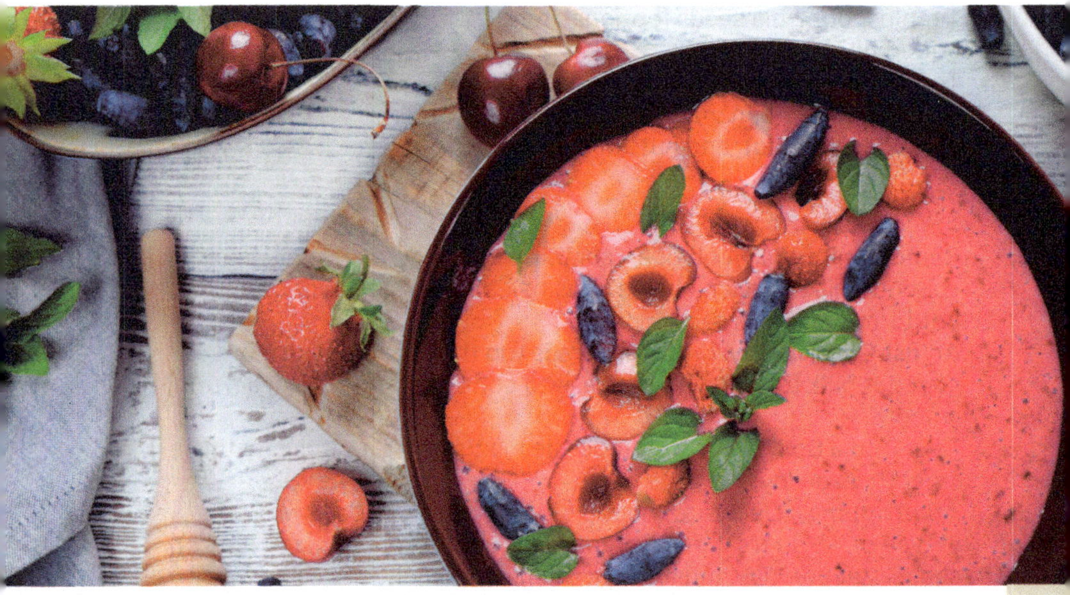

The Berry Bliss Smoothie Bowl is a delightful, nutrient-packed dish that celebrates the vibrant flavors of mixed berries. This recipe is perfect for a quick breakfast, a post-workout recovery, or a refreshing snack any time of the day. Bursting with antioxidants, vitamins, and fiber, this smoothie bowl not only tastes amazing but also supports your overall health. I often prepare this bowl for my family, especially during berry season when the fruits are at their sweetest. The beautiful colors and textures invite creativity, allowing you to personalize your bowl with an array of toppings, making it a fun and engaging way to enjoy healthy eating!

Ingredients

- 1 cup mixed berries (fresh or frozen; strawberries, blueberries, raspberries, and blackberries)
- 1 medium ripe banana (fresh or frozen)
- 1 cup unsweetened almond milk (or any milk of choice)
- 1 tablespoon chia seeds (optional, for added fiber)
- 1 scoop vanilla protein powder (optional, for extra protein)
- Toppings: additional fresh berries, granola, shredded coconut, sliced bananas, nuts, or seeds

Nutrition

Calories	**220**
Protein	**5 g**
Carbohydrates	**38 g**
Sugars	**18 g**
Fats (Total)	**5 g**
Saturated	**1 g**
Unsaturated	**4 g**
Fiber	**6 g**

Instructions

1. **Blend the Base:** In a blender, combine the mixed berries, banana, almond milk, chia seeds (if using), and protein powder (if using). Blend until smooth and creamy.
2. **Adjust Consistency:** If the mixture is too thick, add a little more almond milk to reach your desired consistency. Blend again until fully combined.
3. **Pour into a Bowl:** Pour the smoothie mixture into a bowl, creating a smooth, even layer.
4. **Add Toppings:** Decorate the top of your smoothie bowl with your choice of additional fresh berries, granola, shredded coconut, sliced bananas, and nuts or seeds. Arrange them in a visually appealing manner to make it extra inviting!
5. **Serve Immediately:** Enjoy your Berry Bliss Smoothie Bowl right away for the best flavor and texture.

Nutritionist Tips

- **Berry Selection:** Use a variety of berries to maximize flavor and nutrition. Fresh berries are ideal when in season, but frozen berries work perfectly too and can help create a thicker texture.
- **Customizable Toppings:** Feel free to get creative with your toppings! You can add granola for crunch, nuts for healthy fats, or even a dollop of nut butter for added richness.
- **Experiment with Flavors:** This recipe is highly adaptable; consider adding spinach or kale for an extra nutrient boost without altering the flavor significantly.

Honey-Lavender Frozen Yogurt

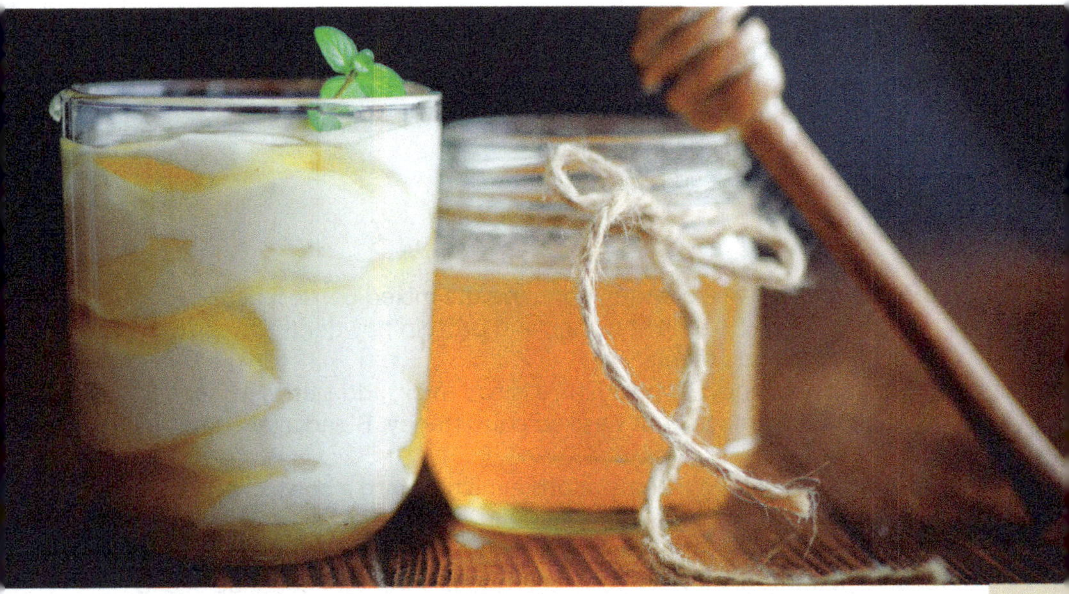

The Honey-Lavender Frozen Yogurt is a delightful, creamy treat that beautifully combines the floral notes of lavender with the natural sweetness of honey. This recipe is perfect for those warm days when you crave something refreshing yet indulgent. The subtle floral aroma of lavender paired with the rich creaminess of yogurt creates a sophisticated dessert that is sure to impress. I love making this frozen yogurt during the spring and summer months, as it captures the essence of the season. It's also a great way to introduce unique flavors to your family while enjoying the health benefits of yogurt. This recipe is simple to prepare and offers a deliciously healthy alternative to traditional ice cream!

Ingredients

- 2 cups plain Greek yogurt (non-fat or full-fat based on preference)
- 1/2 cup honey (adjust to taste; can use agave syrup for a vegan option)
- 1 tablespoon dried culinary lavender (make sure it's food-grade)
- 1 teaspoon pure vanilla extract
- Pinch of salt
- Optional: Additional lavender buds for garnish

Nutrition

Calories	**160**
Protein	**10 g**
Carbohydrates	**25 g**
Sugars	**20 g**
Fats (Total)	**5 g**
Saturated	**2 g**
Unsaturated	**3 g**
Fiber	**0 g**

Instructions

1. **Infuse the Yogurt:** In a small saucepan, combine 1/2 cup of honey and 1/4 cup of water. Add the dried lavender and heat over medium heat until it just begins to simmer. Remove from heat and let it steep for about 15-20 minutes to infuse the flavor.
2. **Strain the Mixture:** After steeping, strain the lavender-infused honey through a fine mesh sieve to remove the lavender buds. Allow the honey to cool slightly.
3. **Combine Ingredients:** In a mixing bowl, whisk together the Greek yogurt, the cooled lavender-infused honey, vanilla extract, and a pinch of salt until smooth and well combined.
4. **Chill the Mixture:** Chill the yogurt mixture in the refrigerator for about 30 minutes to ensure it's cold before freezing.
5. **Freeze the Mixture:** Pour the chilled mixture into your Ninja Creami pint container. Ensure it's filled to the fill line and then freeze for at least 24 hours.

Creami Processing

1. **Creami Processing:** After freezing, remove the pint from the freezer. Place it in your Ninja Creami machine, select the "Ice Cream" function, and process until smooth and creamy.
2. **Serve or Store:** Enjoy immediately for a soft-serve texture or return to the freezer for a firmer consistency. Garnish with additional lavender buds for an elegant touch before serving.

Nutritionist Tips

- **Choosing Lavender:** When selecting lavender, ensure it is culinary-grade and free from pesticides. Dried lavender can often be found in specialty spice shops or online.

Maple Pecan Frozen Yogurt

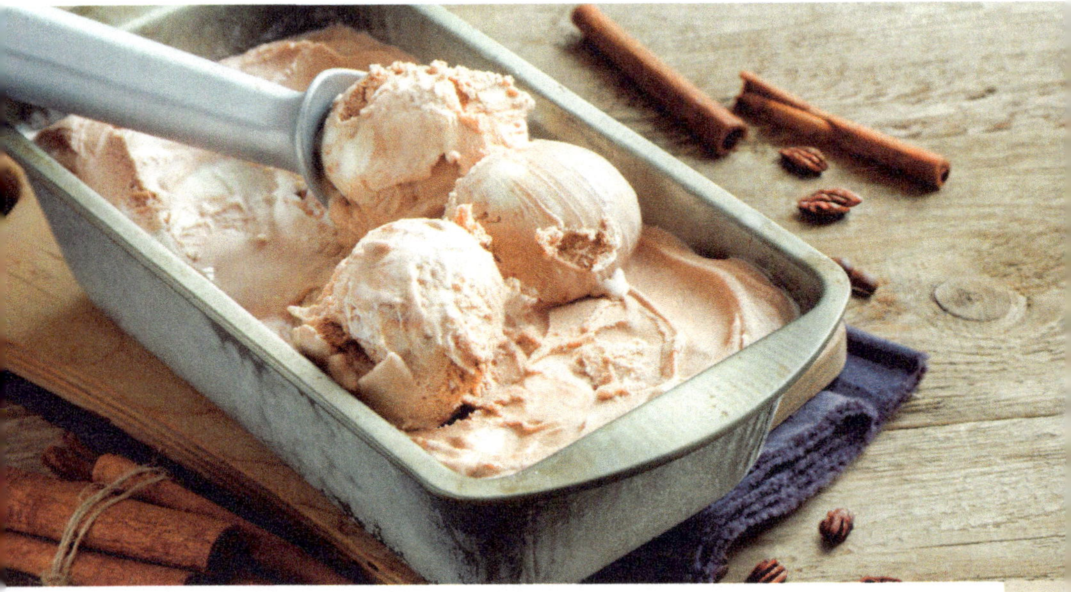

The Maple Pecan Frozen Yogurt is a delightful treat that perfectly combines the rich, nutty flavor of pecans with the warm sweetness of maple syrup. This recipe is a fantastic way to enjoy a creamy dessert that feels indulgent while still being nutritious. I created this frozen yogurt as a healthier alternative to traditional ice cream, ensuring that it satisfies my sweet cravings without the guilt. The crunchy pecans add a wonderful texture that complements the smoothness of the yogurt. This frozen yogurt is perfect for any occasion, whether it's a warm summer day or a cozy winter evening. It's simple to prepare, and you can feel good about serving it to your family!

Ingredients

- 2 cups plain Greek yogurt (non-fat or full-fat based on preference)
- 1/2 cup pure maple syrup (adjust to taste; can use agave syrup for a vegan option)
- 1 teaspoon pure vanilla extract
- 1/2 cup chopped pecans (toasted for extra flavor)
- Pinch of salt

Nutrition

Calories	**210**
Protein	**8 g**
Carbohydrates	**25 g**
Sugars	**12 g**
Fats (Total)	**9 g**
Saturated	**3 g**
Unsaturated	**6 g**
Fiber	**1 g**

Instructions

1. **Combine Ingredients:** In a mixing bowl, whisk together the Greek yogurt, maple syrup, vanilla extract, and a pinch of salt until smooth and well combined.
2. **Toast the Pecans:** If you prefer toasted pecans, place them in a dry skillet over medium heat. Toast for about 3-5 minutes, stirring frequently, until they are fragrant and golden. Remove from heat and let them cool slightly.
3. **Mix in Pecans:** Once the pecans have cooled, fold them into the yogurt mixture, ensuring they are evenly distributed.
4. **Chill the Mixture:** Chill the yogurt mixture in the refrigerator for about 30 minutes to ensure it's cold before freezing.
5. **Freeze the Mixture:** Pour the chilled mixture into your Ninja Creami pint container. Ensure it's filled to the fill line and then freeze for at least 24 hours.

Creami Processing

1. **Creami Processing:** After freezing, remove the pint from the freezer. Place it in your Ninja Creami machine, select the "Ice Cream" function, and process until smooth and creamy.
2. **Serve or Store:** Enjoy immediately for a soft-serve texture or return to the freezer for a firmer consistency. You can garnish with additional chopped pecans or a drizzle of maple syrup before serving.

Nutritionist Tips

- **Maple Syrup Quality:** Choose pure maple syrup for the best flavor and health benefits. Avoid imitation syrups that contain added sugars and artificial flavors.

Creative
LOW-SUGAR DESSERTS

Coconut Lime Popsicles

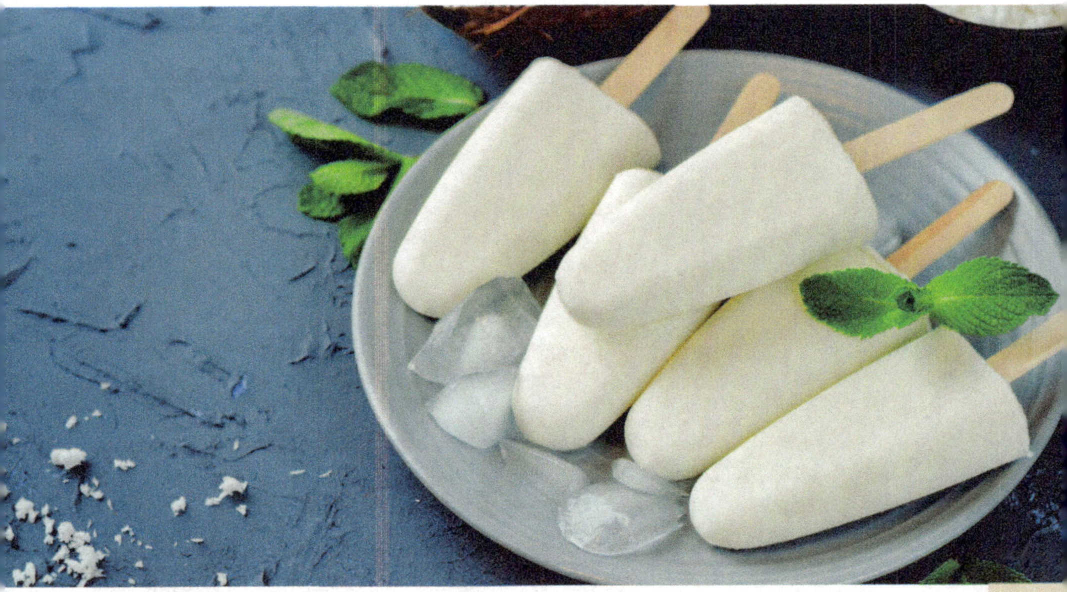

The Coconut Lime Popsicles are a refreshing and zesty treat that transports you straight to a tropical paradise with every bite. The creamy coconut paired with the bright acidity of lime creates a perfect balance of flavors that is both invigorating and satisfying. This recipe is a favorite in my household, especially during the hot summer months when we crave something cool and delicious. Not only are these popsicles easy to make, but they also offer a healthy alternative to store-bought frozen treats, as you can control the ingredients and sweetness. They're a fantastic way to enjoy a guilt-free dessert that's rich in flavor and nutrition!

Ingredients

- 1 can (13.5 oz) full-fat coconut milk (or light coconut milk for a lighter option)
- 1/2 cup unsweetened almond milk (or any milk of choice)
- 1/4 cup honey or maple syrup (adjust to taste; can use sugar-free sweetener for lower sugar)
- Zest of 2 limes
- Juice of 2 limes (about 1/4 cup)
- Pinch of salt

Nutrition

Calories	100
Protein	1 g
Carbohydrates	12 g
Sugars	6 g
Fats (Total)	6 g
Saturated	5 g
Unsaturated	1 g
Fiber	0 g

Instructions

1. **Combine Ingredients:** In a mixing bowl, whisk together the coconut milk, almond milk, honey (or sweetener), lime zest, lime juice, and a pinch of salt until well combined.
2. **Taste and Adjust:** Taste the mixture and adjust sweetness if necessary by adding more honey or maple syrup. Blend again if you make any adjustments.
3. **Pour into Molds:** Pour the mixture evenly into popsicle molds, leaving a little space at the top for expansion. If your molds have lids, insert the sticks according to the manufacturer's instructions.
4. **Freeze:** Place the molds in the freezer and freeze for at least 4-6 hours or until completely solid.
5. **Unmold and Serve:** To remove the popsicles, run warm water over the outside of the molds for a few seconds. Gently pull on the sticks to release the popsicles. Enjoy immediately!

Nutritionist Tips

- **Coconut Milk Selection:** Choose full-fat coconut milk for a creamier texture, but if you prefer a lighter option, light coconut milk works well too.
- **Adjusting Sweetness:** Depending on your preference and the tartness of your limes, you may want to adjust the sweetness. If using sugar-free sweeteners, be sure to check the conversion ratios on the packaging.
- **Flavor Enhancements:** For added flavor, consider mixing in fresh mint leaves or a splash of pineapple juice for a tropical twist.
- **Serving Ideas:** These popsicles are perfect on their own, but you can also serve them alongside fresh fruit or a drizzle of honey for an extra touch.

Green Smoothie Popsicles

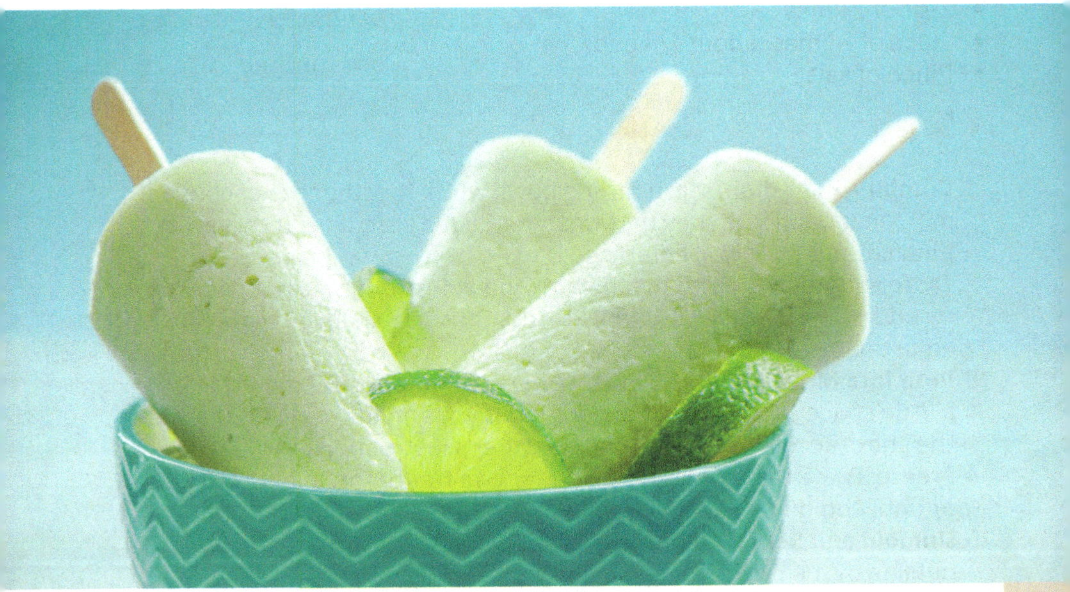

The Green Smoothie Popsicles are a fantastic way to enjoy a nutrient-packed treat while staying cool during those warm days! Bursting with vibrant flavors from fresh fruits and leafy greens, these popsicles provide a deliciously sweet and refreshing option that's perfect for both kids and adults. I created this recipe to help my family get their daily servings of fruits and vegetables in a fun and enjoyable way. They are incredibly versatile, allowing you to mix and match your favorite fruits and greens, making them a delightful addition to your summer routine. These popsicles are not only a hit with my daughter, Emma, but also a great way to introduce new flavors and textures to her diet!

Ingredients

- 1 cup spinach or kale (stems removed)
- 1 ripe banana (fresh or frozen)
- 1 cup unsweetened almond milk (or any milk of choice)
- 1/2 cup pineapple chunks (fresh or frozen)
- 1/2 cup mango chunks (fresh or frozen)
- 1 tablespoon honey or maple syrup (optional, adjust to taste)
- A few ice cubes (optional, for a thicker texture)

Nutrition

Calories	**60**
Protein	**1 g**
Carbohydrates	**14 g**
Sugars	**8 g**
Fats (Total)	**0 g**
Saturated	**0 g**
Unsaturated	**0 g**
Fiber	**2 g**

Instructions

1. **Blend the Mixture:** In a blender, combine the spinach or kale, banana, almond milk, pineapple chunks, mango chunks, and honey (if using). Blend until smooth and creamy. If you prefer a thicker texture, add a few ice cubes and blend again.
2. **Taste and Adjust:** Taste the mixture and adjust sweetness if necessary by adding more honey or maple syrup. Blend again if you make any adjustments.
3. **Prepare the Popsicle Molds:** If you want to add extra fruit pieces, place some chopped fruit at the bottom of each popsicle mold.
4. **Fill the Molds:** Pour the smoothie mixture evenly into the popsicle molds, leaving a little space at the top for expansion.
5. **Insert Sticks:** If your molds have lids, insert the sticks according to the manufacturer's instructions. If not, wait for about 30 minutes until the popsicles start to freeze slightly, then insert the sticks.
6. **Freeze:** Place the molds in the freezer and freeze for at least 4-6 hours or until completely solid.
7. **Unmold and Serve:** To remove the popsicles, run warm water over the outside of the molds for a few seconds. Gently pull on the sticks to release the popsicles. Enjoy immediately!

Nutritionist Tips

- **Choosing Greens:** Spinach is a great option for those new to green smoothies due to its mild flavor. Kale can be used for a more robust taste and additional nutrients.
- **Fruit Variations:** Feel free to mix and match your favorite fruits. Other great additions include kiwi, berries, or even avocado for creaminess.

Peanut Butter Banana Shake

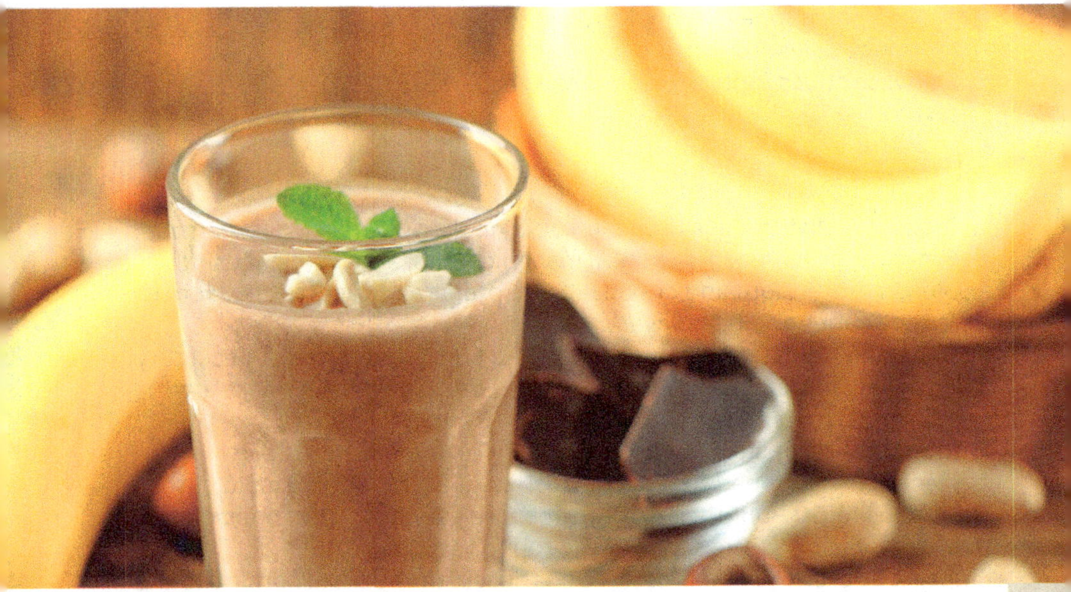

The Peanut Butter Banana Shake is a creamy, indulgent drink that perfectly combines the rich flavor of peanut butter with the natural sweetness of ripe bananas. This shake is not only delicious but also packed with protein and healthy fats, making it an ideal option for breakfast, a post-workout recovery, or a satisfying snack. I love whipping up this shake when I need a quick and nutritious option that keeps me energized throughout the day. It's a favorite in my household, especially with my daughter, Emma, who enjoys the delightful combination of flavors. With just a few simple ingredients, you can create a thick and satisfying shake that feels like a treat!

Ingredients

- 1 cup unsweetened almond milk (or any milk of choice)
- 1 medium ripe banana (fresh or frozen)
- 2 tablespoons natural peanut butter (or almond butter)
- 1 scoop vanilla protein powder (optional, for added protein)
- 1 tablespoon cocoa powder (optional, for a chocolate twist)
- 1 teaspoon honey or maple syrup (optional, adjust to taste)
- Ice cubes (optional, for a thicker texture)

Nutrition

Calories	**300**
Protein	**15 g**
Carbohydrates	**35 g**
Sugars	**15 g**
Fats (Total)	**13 g**
Saturated	**2 g**
Unsaturated	**11 g**
Fiber	**4 g**

Instructions

1. **Combine Ingredients:** In a blender, add the almond milk, banana, peanut butter, protein powder (if using), cocoa powder (if using), honey (if desired), and a handful of ice cubes.
2. **Blend Until Smooth:** Blend on high speed until the mixture is completely smooth and creamy. If it's too thick, you can add more almond milk to reach your desired consistency.
3. **Taste and Adjust:** Taste the shake and adjust sweetness if necessary by adding more honey or maple syrup. Blend again if you make any adjustments.
4. **Serve:** Pour the shake into a glass and enjoy immediately. You can also garnish with a sprinkle of cocoa powder or a few banana slices on top for an extra touch.

Nutritionist Tips

- **Banana Ripeness:** The riper the banana, the sweeter your shake will be. Look for bananas with brown spots for maximum sweetness.
- **Nut Butter Alternatives:** If you have nut allergies, consider using sunflower seed butter or tahini as a substitute for peanut butter.
- **Chocolate Variation:** For a chocolatey flavor, the addition of cocoa powder works beautifully with the peanut butter and banana. This creates a delicious chocolate peanut butter shake that feels indulgent.
- **Add-Ins:** Feel free to add a scoop of chia seeds or flaxseeds for extra fiber and omega-3 fatty acids, or toss in a handful of spinach for added nutrients without changing the flavor.

Spinach Pineapple Smoothie

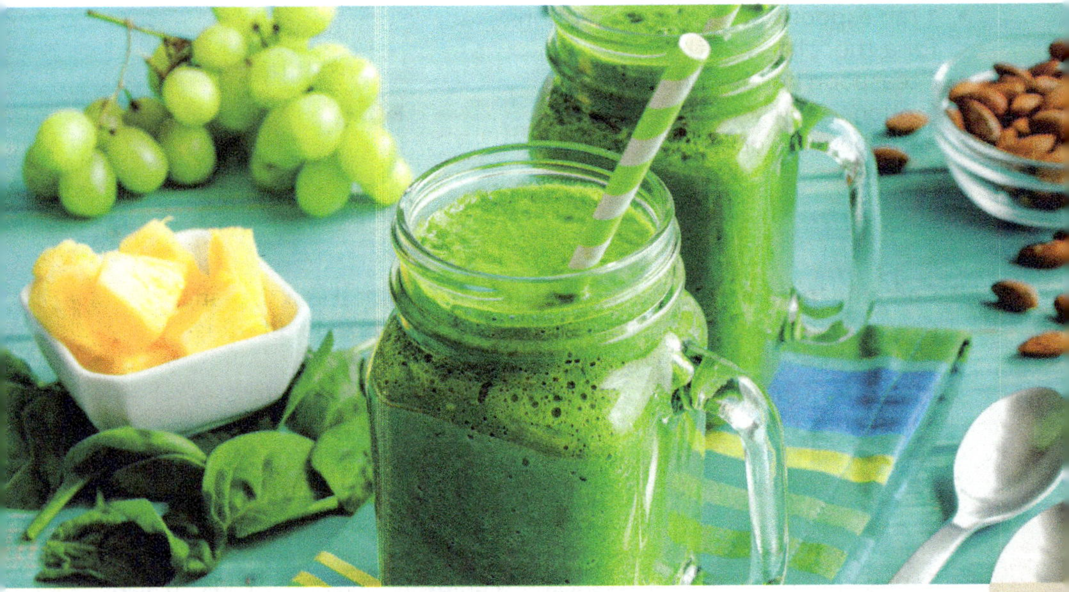

The Spinach Pineapple Smoothie is a refreshing and vibrant drink that perfectly combines the tropical sweetness of pineapple with the nutrient-dense goodness of spinach. This smoothie is not only delicious but also packed with vitamins and minerals, making it an excellent choice for breakfast or a post-workout boost. I created this recipe to help my family enjoy more greens in a fun and tasty way. The pineapple masks the flavor of the spinach beautifully, making it a favorite among both kids and adults. It's a simple, quick recipe that's perfect for busy mornings or anytime you need a healthy pick-me-up!

Ingredients

- 1 cup fresh spinach (stems removed)
- 1 cup frozen pineapple chunks (or fresh pineapple, chopped)
- 1 medium banana (fresh or frozen)
- 1 cup unsweetened almond milk (or any milk of choice)
- 1 tablespoon chia seeds (optional, for added fiber and omega-3s)
- 1 teaspoon honey or maple syrup (optional, adjust to taste)
- Ice cubes (optional, for a thicker texture)

Nutrition

Calories	**180**
Protein	**4 g**
Carbohydrates	**36 g**
Sugars	**20 g**
Fats (Total)	**3 g**
Saturated	**0.5 g**
Unsaturated	**2.5 g**
Fiber	**5 g**

Instructions

1. **Combine Ingredients:** In a blender, add the spinach, frozen pineapple, banana, almond milk, chia seeds (if using), and honey (if desired). If you prefer a thicker smoothie, add a handful of ice cubes.
2. **Blend Until Smooth:** Blend on high speed until the mixture is completely smooth and creamy. If it's too thick, you can add more almond milk to reach your desired consistency.
3. **Taste and Adjust:** Taste the smoothie and adjust sweetness if necessary by adding more honey or maple syrup. Blend again if you make any adjustments.
4. **Serve:** Pour the smoothie into a glass and enjoy immediately. For an extra touch, you can garnish with a slice of pineapple or a sprinkle of chia seeds on top.

Nutritionist Tips

- **Choosing Spinach:** Fresh spinach is preferred for its mild flavor, but you can also use baby spinach or even kale for added nutrients. If using frozen spinach, ensure it's thawed and drained before blending.
- **Fruit Variations:** Feel free to experiment with other tropical fruits like mango or banana for added sweetness and flavor. The combination of fruits can significantly change the taste, so have fun with it!
- **Boost Nutrition:** For an extra nutrient boost, consider adding a scoop of protein powder or a tablespoon of nut butter to the smoothie.

Chia Seed Pudding with Fresh Fruits

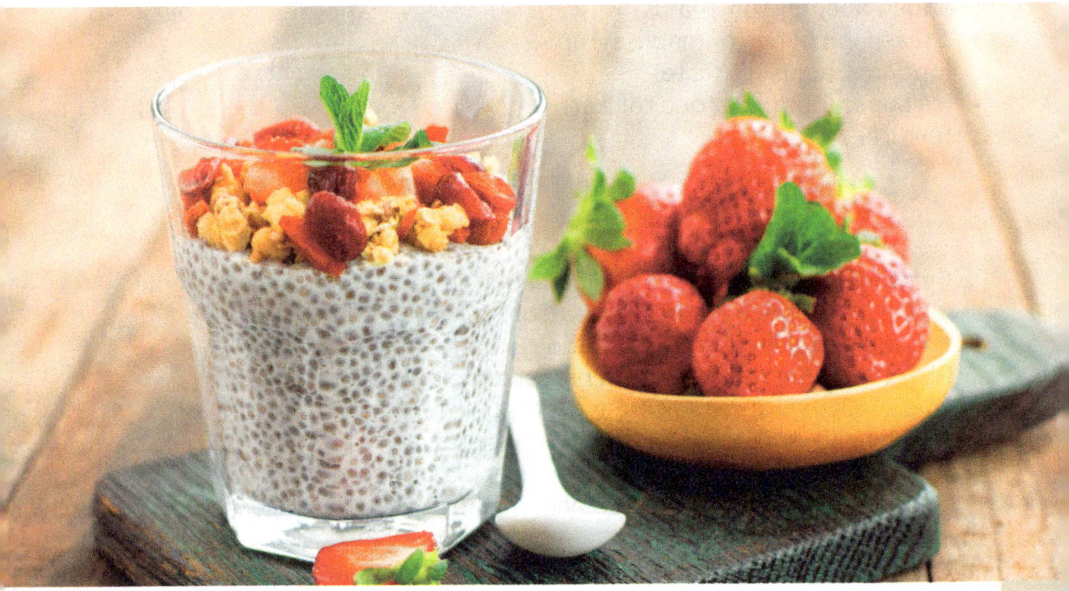

The Chia Seed Pudding with Fresh Fruits is a simple yet delicious treat that highlights the nutritious power of chia seeds. This pudding is not only rich in omega-3 fatty acids and fiber but also incredibly versatile, allowing you to customize it with your favorite fruits and toppings. I love preparing this pudding as a quick breakfast option or a satisfying snack, especially during busy mornings. The combination of creamy chia pudding topped with vibrant, fresh fruits creates a beautiful and flavorful dish that both kids and adults will enjoy. It's a fantastic way to incorporate more whole foods into your diet while indulging in a delightful dessert!

Ingredients

- 1/2 cup chia seeds
- 2 cups unsweetened almond milk (or any milk of choice)
- 1/4 cup honey or maple syrup (adjust to taste; can use sugar-free sweetener for lower sugar)
- 1 teaspoon pure vanilla extract
- Pinch of salt
- Fresh fruits for topping (such as berries, sliced bananas, mango, or kiwi)
- Optional toppings: nuts, seeds, coconut flakes, or granola

Nutrition

Calories	**180**
Protein	**5 g**
Carbohydrates	**25 g**
Sugars	**10 g**
Fats (Total)	**7 g**
Saturated	**1 g**
Unsaturated	**6 g**
Fiber	**8 g**

Instructions

1. **Combine Ingredients:** In a mixing bowl, whisk together the chia seeds, almond milk, honey (or sweetener), vanilla extract, and a pinch of salt until well combined.
2. **Let It Sit:** Allow the mixture to sit for about 5-10 minutes, then whisk again to prevent the chia seeds from clumping together. This step is crucial for achieving a smooth texture.
3. **Refrigerate:** Cover the bowl or transfer the mixture to individual serving jars and refrigerate for at least 4 hours or overnight. The chia seeds will absorb the liquid and thicken into a pudding-like consistency.
4. **Serve:** Once the pudding has thickened, give it a good stir before serving. If it's too thick, you can add a splash of milk to reach your desired consistency.
5. **Add Fresh Fruits:** Top the chia pudding with your choice of fresh fruits. Get creative with your toppings, layering different fruits for a colorful presentation.
6. **Optional Toppings:** For added texture, consider sprinkling nuts, seeds, coconut flakes, or granola on top before enjoying.

Nutritionist Tips

- **Chia Seed Benefits:** Chia seeds are a fantastic source of fiber and healthy fats, making this pudding not only filling but also beneficial for digestion and heart health.

Layered Yogurt Parfait

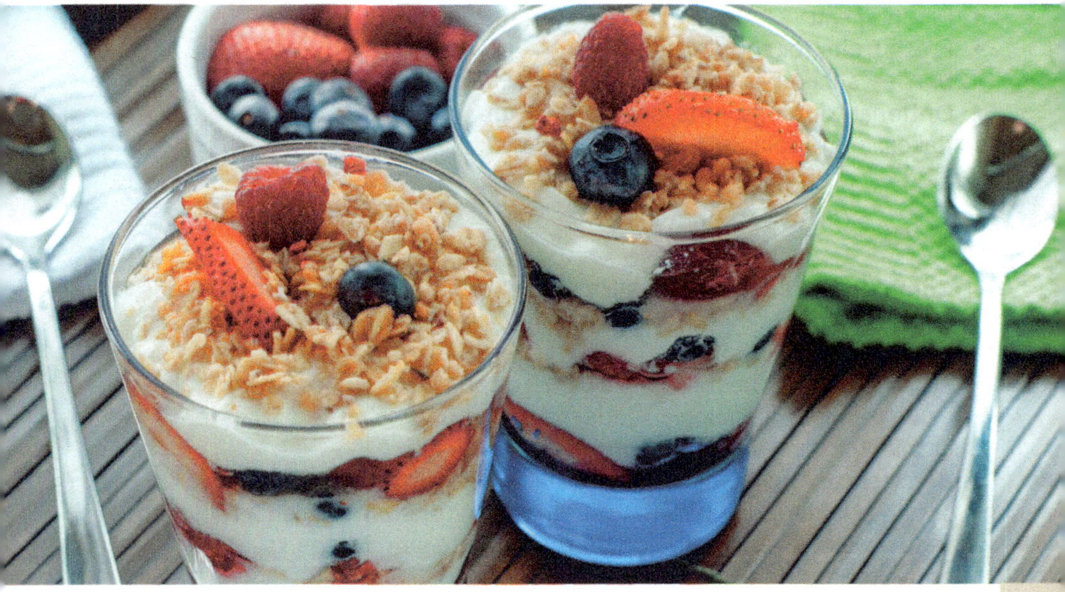

The Layered Yogurt Parfait is a delightful and visually appealing treat that brings together creamy yogurt, vibrant fruits, and crunchy granola in a harmonious blend. This recipe is perfect for breakfast, a snack, or even dessert, allowing you to enjoy the deliciousness of wholesome ingredients while balancing flavors and textures. I love preparing this parfait for my family, especially because it's easy to customize with our favorite fruits and toppings. It's a fantastic way to get the kids involved in the kitchen, as they can help layer the ingredients and create their own unique creations. This parfait is not only nutritious but also a beautiful addition to any meal!

Ingredients

- 2 cups plain Greek yogurt (non-fat or full-fat based on preference)
- 1 cup mixed fresh berries (such as strawberries, blueberries, raspberries, and blackberries)
- 1/2 cup granola (store-bought or homemade)
- 2 tablespoons honey or maple syrup (optional, adjust to taste)
- 1 teaspoon vanilla extract (optional)
- Additional toppings: sliced almonds, chia seeds, or shredded coconut (optional)

Nutrition

Calories	**180**
Protein	**10 g**
Carbohydrates	**25 g**
Sugars	**10 g**
Fats (Total)	**5 g**
Saturated	**2 g**
Unsaturated	**3 g**
Fiber	**3 g**

Instructions

1. **Prepare the Yogurt:** In a mixing bowl, combine the Greek yogurt, honey (if using), and vanilla extract (if using). Stir well until smooth and creamy.
2. **Prepare the Fruit:** Wash and slice the fresh berries as needed. If using larger fruits like strawberries, slice them into smaller pieces for layering.
3. **Layer the Parfait:** In serving glasses or bowls, start by adding a layer of the yogurt mixture at the bottom. Follow with a layer of mixed berries, then add a layer of granola. Repeat the layers until the glasses are filled, finishing with a layer of yogurt on top.
4. **Top and Garnish:** If desired, garnish the top with additional berries, a sprinkle of granola, and any optional toppings such as sliced almonds or shredded coconut for added flavor and texture.
5. **Serve Immediately:** Enjoy your layered yogurt parfait right away for the best flavor and texture. If preparing in advance, keep the granola separate until ready to serve to maintain its crunch.

Nutritionist Tips

- **Yogurt Selection:** Opt for plain Greek yogurt for its high protein content and creamy texture. You can also use plant-based yogurt if you prefer a dairy-free option.
- **Granola Choices:** Choose a granola that is low in added sugars and high in whole grains. Making your own granola allows you to control the ingredients and sweetness.

FAMILY FRIENDLY RECIPES

Chocolate Chip Cookie Dough Ice Cream

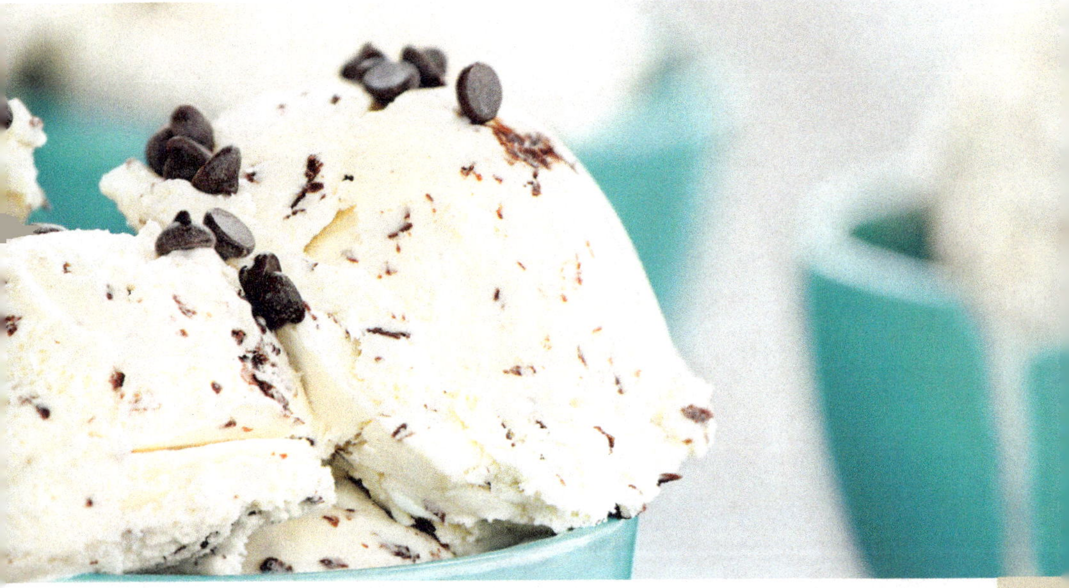

The Chocolate Chip Cookie Dough Ice Cream is a delightful combination of rich, creamy ice cream and indulgent cookie dough pieces that brings the classic dessert to a whole new level. This recipe captures the nostalgia of freshly baked cookies while providing a healthier, guilt-free version that you can enjoy anytime. I developed this recipe to satisfy my family's love for cookie dough and ice cream, allowing us to indulge without compromising our health goals. The homemade cookie dough is safe to eat raw, and the creamy base complements the sweet, chewy bites perfectly. It's a fun addition to any gathering and a treat that will delight both kids and adults alike!

Ingredients

For the Ice Cream Base:

- 2 cups heavy cream (or coconut cream for a dairy-free option)
- 1 cup whole milk (or almond milk for a dairy-free option)
- 1/2 cup granulated sugar or your preferred sweetener (adjust to taste; can use agave syrup or erythritol for lower sugar)
- 1 teaspoon pure vanilla extract
- Pinch of salt

For the Cookie Dough:

- 1/2 cup all-purpose flour (or gluten-free flour for a gluten-free option)
- 1/4 cup unsalted butter, softened (or coconut oil for dairy-free)
- 1/4 cup brown sugar (or coconut sugar for a lower glycemic option)
- 2 tablespoons granulated sugar (or low-carb sweetener)
- 1 teaspoon vanilla extract
- 1/8 teaspoon salt
- 1/4 cup mini chocolate chips

Nutrition

Calories	**300**
Protein	**4 g**
Carbohydrates	**30 g**
Sugars	**15 g**
Fats (Total)	**18 g**
Saturated	**10 g**
Unsaturated	**8 g**
Fiber	**1 g**

Instructions

Prepare the Ice Cream Base:

1. **Combine Ingredients:** In a medium saucepan, whisk together the heavy cream, whole milk, sugar (or sweetener), vanilla extract, and a pinch of salt over medium heat until smooth and well combined.
2. **Cool the Mixture:** Allow the mixture to cool to room temperature. For quicker cooling, transfer it to a bowl and refrigerate for about 30 minutes.
3. **Freeze the Base:** Pour the cooled mixture into your Ninja Creami pint container. Ensure it's filled to the fill line and then freeze for at least 24 hours.

Instructions

Prepare the Cookie Dough:

1. **Mix Cookie Dough Ingredients:** In a mixing bowl, cream together the softened butter, brown sugar, granulated sugar, vanilla extract, and salt until smooth. Gradually mix in the flour until combined, and then fold in the mini chocolate chips.
2. **Form Cookie Dough Balls:** Form the cookie dough into small balls or chunks. Place them on a parchment-lined baking sheet and refrigerate while you prepare the ice cream.

Creami Processing:

1. **Creami Processing:** After freezing the ice cream base, remove it from the freezer. Place it in your Ninja Creami machine, select the "Ice Cream" function, and process until smooth.
2. **Add Cookie Dough:** Gently fold in the chilled cookie dough pieces into the ice cream after processing.
3. **Serve or Store:** Enjoy immediately for a soft-serve texture or return to the freezer for a firmer consistency. For an extra treat, drizzle with chocolate syrup or top with more mini chocolate chips before serving.

Nutritionist Tips

- **Flour Safety:** To make the cookie dough safe to eat raw, you can heat-treat the flour by baking it at 350°F (175°C) for about 5 minutes to kill any potential bacteria.
- **Sweetener Options:** If you prefer a lower sugar version, consider using a sugar-free sweetener like erythritol or a blend of sweeteners to achieve the desired sweetness.
- **Texture Enhancements:** For added crunch, you can incorporate chopped nuts into the cookie dough or add a sprinkle of sea salt on top before serving for a sweet and salty contrast.

Hi There!

I hope you are enjoying my book so far. I would really appreciate it if you could leave a quick review on Amazon.

Just simply scan the code below using your mobile phone's camera, or you can enter the link below on our web browser.

https://swiy.com/ReviewCreami2

Thanks a lot!

- Clara

Fruity Pebbles Ice Cream

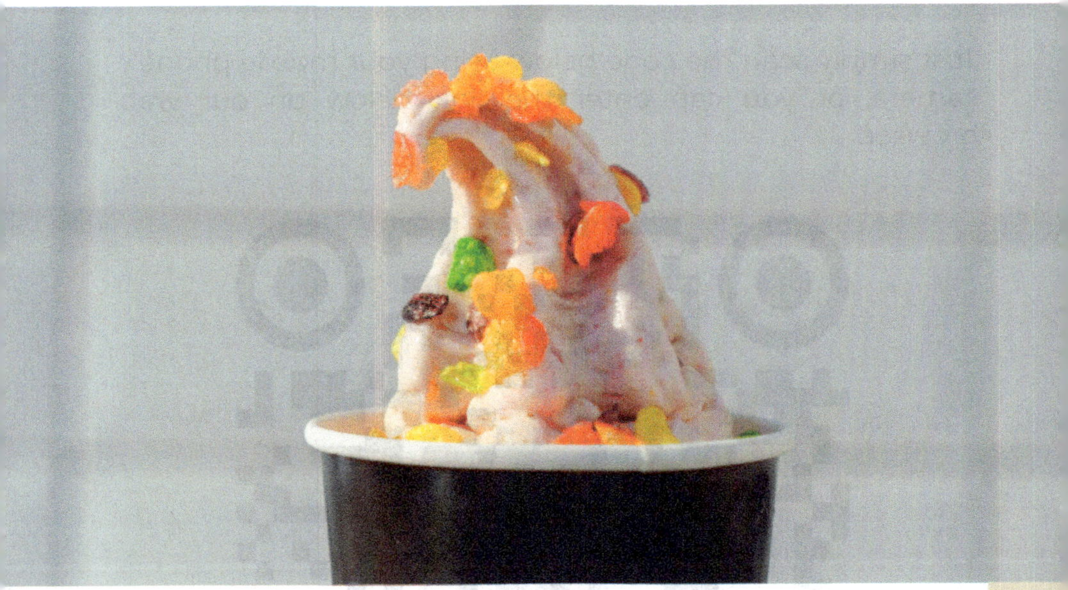

The Fruity Pebbles Ice Cream is a fun and colorful treat that brings a nostalgic twist to your dessert experience! Inspired by the beloved cereal, this ice cream captures the vibrant flavors and playful crunch of Fruity Pebbles, making it a hit with both kids and adults alike. I created this recipe to celebrate the joy of childhood favorites while ensuring it remains a guilt-free indulgence. The combination of creamy vanilla ice cream with the fruity cereal adds a delightful texture and flavor that is perfect for warm days or festive celebrations. It's a simple recipe that can be made in no time, and it's sure to bring smiles to your family's faces!

Ingredients

- 2 cups heavy cream (or coconut cream for a dairy-free option)
- 1 cup whole milk (or almond milk for a dairy-free option)
- 1/2 cup granulated sugar or your preferred sweetener (adjust to taste; can use agave syrup or erythritol for lower sugar)
- 1 teaspoon pure vanilla extract
- Pinch of salt
- 1 cup Fruity Pebbles cereal (plus extra for garnish)

Nutrition

Calories	**220**
Protein	**3 g**
Carbohydrates	**28 g**
Sugars	**12 g**
Fats (Total)	**12 g**
Saturated	**7 g**
Unsaturated	**5 g**
Fiber	**0 g**

Instructions

1. **Combine Ingredients:** In a medium saucepan, whisk together the heavy cream, whole milk, sugar (or sweetener), vanilla extract, and a pinch of salt over medium heat until smooth and well combined.
2. **Cool the Mixture:** Allow the mixture to cool to room temperature. For quicker cooling, transfer it to a bowl and refrigerate for about 30 minutes.
3. **Freeze the Base:** Pour the cooled mixture into your Ninja Creami pint container. Ensure it's filled to the fill line and then freeze for at least 24 hours.

Creami Processing

1. **Creami Processing:** After freezing, remove the pint from the freezer. Place it in your Ninja Creami machine, select the "Ice Cream" function, and process until smooth and creamy.
2. **Add Fruity Pebbles:** Gently fold in the Fruity Pebbles cereal after processing to maintain their crunch.
3. **Serve or Store:** Enjoy immediately for a soft-serve texture or return to the freezer for a firmer consistency. For an extra fun touch, garnish with additional Fruity Pebbles on top before serving.

Nutritionist Tips

- **Cereal Alternatives:** If you want to experiment with flavors, consider using other colorful cereals or even homemade granola to create unique variations of this recipe.

Frozen Yogurt Bark

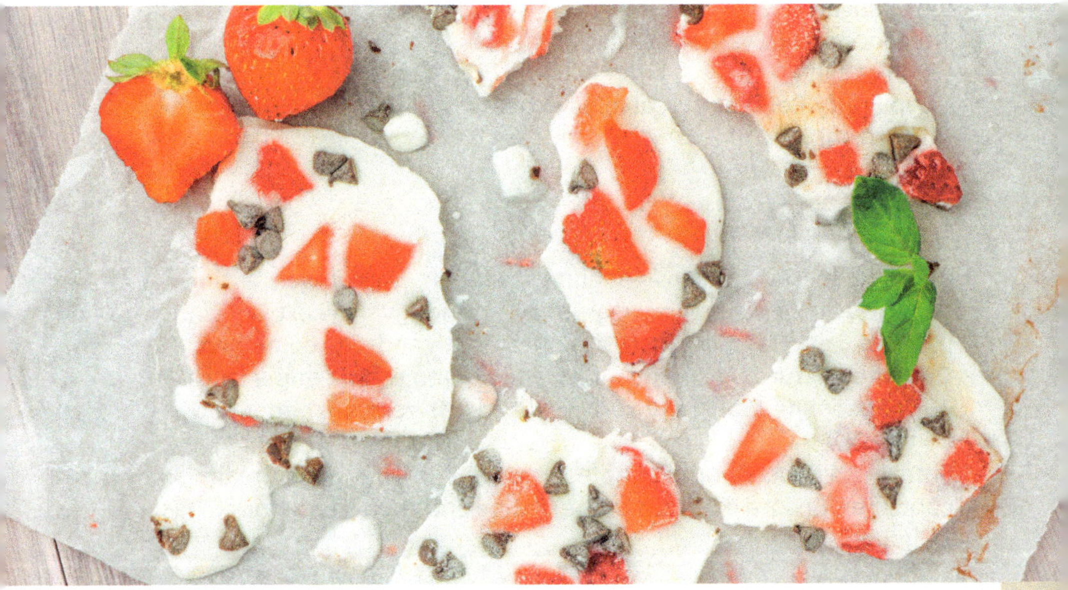

The Frozen Yogurt Bark is a delightful and healthy treat that's perfect for snacking, dessert, or even breakfast! This recipe is incredibly versatile and can be customized with your favorite toppings, making it a fun way to enjoy a variety of flavors and textures. I created this frozen yogurt bark to offer a refreshing alternative to traditional ice cream, providing a nutritious option that my family loves. It's easy to prepare and can be made ahead of time, making it a convenient choice for busy days. The combination of creamy yogurt and fresh fruits creates a beautiful and satisfying dessert that everyone will enjoy!

Ingredients

- 2 cups plain Greek yogurt (non-fat or full-fat based on preference)
- 2 tablespoons honey or maple syrup (adjust to taste; can use sugar-free sweetener for lower sugar)
- 1 teaspoon pure vanilla extract
- 1 cup mixed fresh fruits (such as strawberries, blueberries, raspberries, and kiwi)
- Optional toppings: chopped nuts, shredded coconut, or granola

Nutrition

Calories	**100**
Protein	**6 g**
Carbohydrates	**15 g**
Sugars	**7 g**
Fats (Total)	**2 g**
Saturated	**1 g**
Unsaturated	**1 g**
Fiber	**1 g**

Instructions

1. **Prepare the Yogurt Mixture:** In a mixing bowl, combine the Greek yogurt, honey (or sweetener), and vanilla extract. Stir until well mixed and smooth.
2. **Line the Baking Sheet:** Line a baking sheet or a shallow dish with parchment paper, ensuring it covers the bottom completely for easy removal later.
3. **Spread the Yogurt:** Pour the yogurt mixture onto the prepared baking sheet. Use a spatula to spread it evenly to about 1/4 inch thick.
4. **Add Fresh Fruits:** Evenly distribute the mixed fresh fruits over the yogurt layer, pressing them down slightly to ensure they stick. If desired, sprinkle with any optional toppings like chopped nuts or shredded coconut.
5. **Freeze:** Place the baking sheet in the freezer and freeze for at least 4 hours or until the yogurt is completely firm.
6. **Break into Pieces:** Once fully frozen, remove the bark from the freezer. Lift the parchment paper to remove the yogurt bark from the baking sheet and break it into pieces of your desired size.
7. **Store:** Store the frozen yogurt bark pieces in an airtight container in the freezer for up to two weeks.

Nutritionist Tips

- **Granola Choices:** Choose a granola that is low in added sugars and high in whole grains. Making your own granola allows you to control the ingredients and sweetness.

Apple Cinnamon Frozen Treats

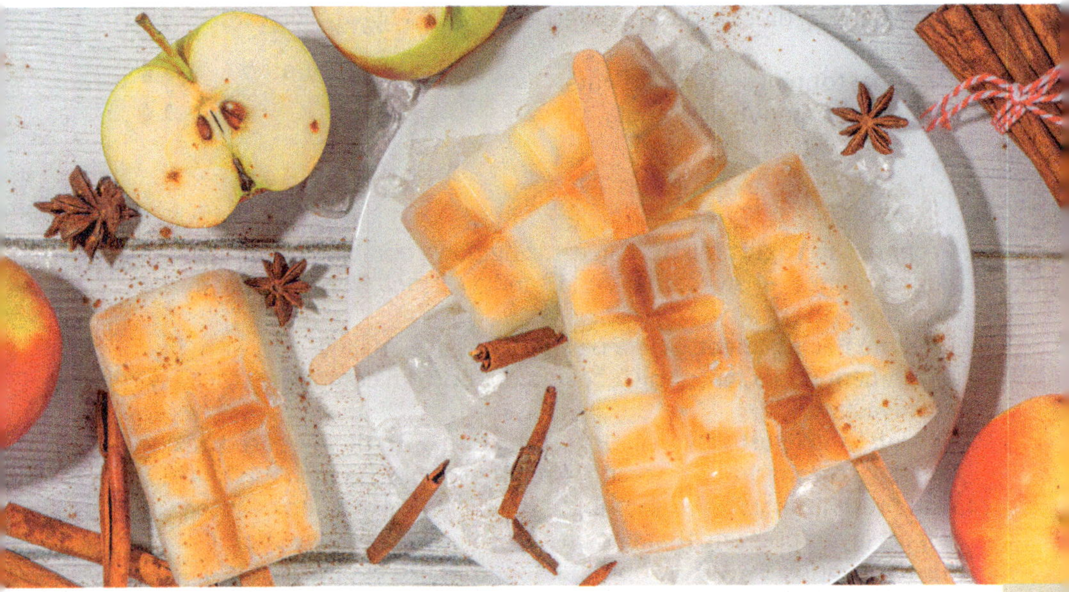

These Apple Cinnamon Frozen Treats are a delightful way to enjoy the comforting flavors of apple pie in a healthy, frozen form. Perfect for warm days or as a nutritious dessert option, these treats are packed with the sweetness of apples and the warm spice of cinnamon. I developed this recipe to provide my family with a fun and easy way to enjoy fruit while keeping it healthy. They're simple to prepare and can be made in advance, making them a convenient choice for busy days. These frozen treats are not only refreshing but also a great way to introduce seasonal flavors to your dessert repertoire!

Ingredients

- 2 cups unsweetened applesauce (store-bought or homemade)
- 1 medium ripe banana, mashed
- 1 teaspoon ground cinnamon
- 1 tablespoon honey or maple syrup (optional, adjust to taste)
- A pinch of salt
- Optional: 1/4 cup chopped nuts (such as walnuts or pecans) for added texture

Nutrition

Calories	70
Protein	1 g
Carbohydrates	17 g
Sugars	0 g
Fats (Total)	0.5 g
Saturated	0 g
Unsaturated	0.5 g
Fiber	2 g

Instructions

1. **Combine Ingredients:** In a mixing bowl, combine the applesauce, mashed banana, ground cinnamon, honey (if using), and a pinch of salt. Mix well until all the ingredients are thoroughly combined.
2. **Add Optional Nuts:** If you're using chopped nuts, fold them into the mixture for added crunch and flavor.
3. **Prepare the Molds:** Pour the mixture into popsicle molds, filling them to the top. If your molds have lids, insert the sticks according to the manufacturer's instructions.
4. **Freeze:** Place the molds in the freezer and freeze for at least 4-6 hours or until completely solid.
5. **Unmold and Serve:** To remove the frozen treats, run warm water over the outside of the molds for a few seconds. Gently pull on the sticks to release the frozen treats. Enjoy immediately!

Nutritionist Tips

- **Applesauce Choice:** For the best flavor, use unsweetened applesauce. You can also make your own by cooking down peeled and diced apples until soft, then blending them into a smooth sauce.
- **Sweetener Adjustments:** Depending on the sweetness of your applesauce and banana, you may choose to adjust the sweetness by adding more honey or maple syrup. Taste the mixture before freezing to ensure it meets your preference.
- **Flavor Variations:** Feel free to experiment with additional spices like nutmeg or ginger for a more complex flavor profile. You can also add a dash of vanilla extract for extra depth.
- **Serving Suggestions:** These frozen treats can be enjoyed on their own or served alongside Greek yogurt for a delicious snack or dessert.

MEAL PREP AND PLANNING

Quick Meal Prep Tips for Busy Families

In our fast-paced lives, effective meal prep can be a lifesaver, particularly when it comes to maintaining a healthy diet. Here are some practical tips specifically designed to help busy families streamline their meal prep while incorporating nutritious frozen treats into their routine:

Schedule Weekly Prep Time
Designate a specific day each week for meal prep. This could be a weekend day when you have a bit more time, or a weekday evening when you can prepare for the days ahead. Planning your meals in advance can help you stay organized and make healthier choices.

Batch Cooking
Prepare larger quantities of key ingredients like smoothie bases, yogurt mixtures, and ice cream bases. This allows you to mix and match components throughout the week, saving time while ensuring variety in your meals.

Utilize Freezer-Friendly Recipes
Take advantage of the Ninja Creami by preparing larger batches of frozen treats and storing them in individual portions. This way, you can quickly grab a nutritious snack or dessert when you need it.

Keep It Simple
Focus on straightforward recipes that require minimal ingredients and preparation time. The easier the recipe, the more likely you are to stick with your meal prep routine.

Involve the Family

Make meal prep a family activity! Get your kids involved by allowing them to help wash fruits, measure ingredients, or layer ingredients in jars. This not only teaches valuable skills but also makes healthy eating a fun and engaging experience.

Plan for Snacks

Don't forget to include healthy snacks in your meal prep. Prepare protein-packed energy bites, yogurt parfaits, or fruit and nut mixes to have on hand for quick, nutritious options.

Organize Your Kitchen

Keep your pantry stocked with essential ingredients for quick access during meal prep. Having a clean and organized kitchen can make the process smoother and more enjoyable.

How to Create Your Own Healthy Treats Meal Plans

Creating a meal plan that incorporates healthy treats can help you meet your nutritional goals while keeping your family satisfied. Here's how to get started:

1. **Assess Nutritional Needs:** Begin by determining the nutritional requirements for your family members based on their age, activity level, and health goals. This will help you tailor your meal plan to ensure everyone is getting the nutrients they need.

2. **Incorporate Protein-Rich Ingredients:** When planning your meals and snacks, focus on incorporating protein-rich ingredients. This can include yogurt, protein powders, nuts, seeds, and legumes. The recipes in this cookbook will guide you in creating treats that are high in protein and satisfying.

3. **Plan Balanced Meals:** Each meal should include a source of protein, healthy fats, and carbohydrates. For example, a balanced meal might consist of grilled chicken, quinoa, and roasted vegetables, while a nutritious snack could be a smoothie made with Greek yogurt, fruits, and protein powder.

4. **Create a Weekly Menu:** Write down your meals for the week, including breakfast, lunch, dinner, and snacks. This structured approach helps you stay organized and ensures you're incorporating enough protein and variety into your family's diet.

5. **Make a Grocery List:** Based on your meal plan, create a detailed grocery list that includes all the ingredients you'll need. This will make shopping more efficient and help you avoid impulse buys.

6. **Prep Ahead:** Cook and prepare key components in advance, such as smoothie bases, ice cream mixtures, and snack options. Having these ready to go will save time during busy weekdays and make it easier to stick to your healthy eating goals.

7. **Be Flexible:** Life can be unpredictable, so be prepared to adjust your meal plan as needed. If you have leftovers from one meal, incorporate them into another day's meals to minimize waste and save time.

By following these meal prep tips and strategies for creating healthy treats meal plans, you can simplify your cooking process and ensure that your family enjoys nutritious meals throughout the week. Let's dive into the exciting recipes that will help you maximize your health while indulging in delicious frozen treats!

SHOPPING
MADE SIMPLE

Essential Ingredients to Stock for Healthy Frozen Treats

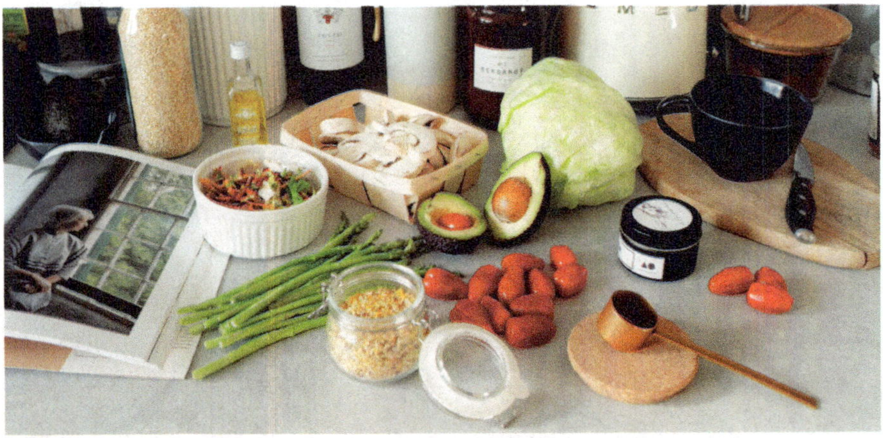

To create delicious and nutritious frozen treats, it's essential to have a well-stocked kitchen with key ingredients that support your health goals. Here's a list of must-have items you should consider having on hand:

Dairy and Dairy Alternatives

- Heavy Cream or Coconut Cream: These provide a rich base for making creamy ice creams.
- Greek Yogurt: A versatile ingredient that adds creaminess and protein to your frozen desserts. Opt for plain, unsweetened varieties to avoid added sugars.
- Milk Options: Unsweetened almond milk, coconut milk, or oat milk can be used as bases for smoothies or frozen treats.

Sweeteners

- Natural Sweeteners: Honey, maple syrup, or agave syrup can enhance the flavor of your recipes. For lower-sugar options, consider using erythritol, stevia, or monk fruit sweetener.
- Granulated Sugar: A staple for traditional recipes, though it's wise to use it sparingly.

Fruits

- Fresh and Frozen Fruits: Berries, bananas, mangoes, and peaches are great for adding natural sweetness and flavor to your frozen treats. Frozen fruits are convenient for smoothies and sorbets.

Protein Sources

- Protein Powder: Whether it's whey or plant-based, protein powder is an easy way to boost the nutritional content of your treats.
- Nut Butters: Almond butter, peanut butter, and sunflower seed butter provide healthy fats and protein.

Nuts and Seeds

- Nuts: Almonds, walnuts, pecans, and pistachios can add crunch and healthy fats. They can be used in recipes or as toppings.
- Seeds: Chia seeds and flaxseeds are excellent sources of fiber and omega-3 fatty acids, perfect for incorporating into smoothies or frozen desserts.

Flavorings and Spices

- Extracts: Vanilla extract, almond extract, and peppermint extract can enhance the flavor of your desserts.
- Spices: Ground cinnamon, nutmeg, and ginger add warmth and depth to many recipes.

Grains

- Oats: Rolled oats are great for adding texture to recipes and can be used in granola or as a base for energy bites.

Where to Find

Nutritious Ingredients

Finding high-quality, nutritious ingredients is essential for preparing healthy frozen treats. Here are some tips on where to shop for these essential items:

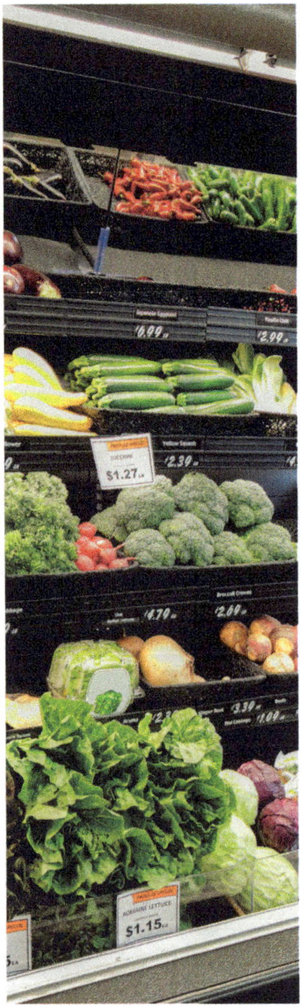

1. **Local Grocery Stores:** Most grocery stores carry a variety of healthy ingredients, including fresh produce, dairy alternatives, and pantry staples. Look for organic options when possible to maximize nutritional benefits.
2. **Health Food Stores:** These stores often have a wider selection of specialty items, such as protein powders, non-dairy yogurts, and organic grains. They can also provide unique ingredients that may not be available at regular grocery stores.
3. **Farmers' Markets:** Fresh, seasonal produce can often be found at local farmers' markets. This is a great way to support local agriculture while obtaining high-quality fruits and vegetables for your recipes.
4. **Online Retailers:** Consider purchasing bulk items like nuts, seeds, and specialty ingredients from reputable online retailers. This is a convenient option for stocking up on pantry staples.
5. **Warehouse Clubs:** Stores like Costco or Sam's Club can provide bulk options for many healthy ingredients at a lower price point, making it easy to stock up on essentials for your frozen treats.

TIPS FOR SUCCESS

Navigating Social Situations with Healthy Treats

Maintaining healthy eating habits can be particularly challenging in social situations where indulgent foods often take center stage. However, with some planning and strategies, you can enjoy gatherings while staying true to your health goals. Here are some tips to help you navigate social situations with confidence:

- **Bring Your Own Treats**: If you're attending a party or gathering, consider bringing a healthy dessert or snack that you can enjoy. This not only ensures you have something nutritious to indulge in but also introduces others to delicious healthy options.

- **Make Smart Choices:** When faced with a buffet or dessert table, take a moment to assess your options. Look for healthier choices like fruit salads, yogurt parfaits, or dark chocolate. If you choose to indulge, opt for smaller portions to keep your overall intake balanced.

- **Communicate Your Goals:** Don't hesitate to share your dietary preferences or goals with friends and family. Many people are supportive and will appreciate your commitment to healthy eating. You may even inspire them to join you in making healthier choices!

- **Stay Mindful:** Practice mindful eating by savoring each bite and enjoying the flavors of the food. This can help you feel satisfied with smaller portions and reduce the likelihood of overindulging.

Involving Family in the Kitchen:

Fun Activities for Kids

Cooking together is a wonderful way to bond as a family and teach children valuable skills about healthy eating. Here are some fun activities to involve your kids in the kitchen:

- **Recipe Selection:** Let your children help choose recipes from this cookbook. Involving them in the decision-making process makes them more excited to participate in the preparation.

- **Ingredient Prep:** Allow kids to wash fruits, measure ingredients, and mix mixtures. This hands-on involvement fosters confidence and a sense of accomplishment.

- **Creative Presentation:** Encourage kids to get creative with the presentation of dishes. They can help arrange toppings on smoothie bowls or decorate popsicles, making healthy eating more fun.

- **Theme Nights:** Host themed cooking nights where each family member can choose a cuisine or type of treat to prepare together. This not only encourages creativity but also exposes kids to different cultures and flavors.

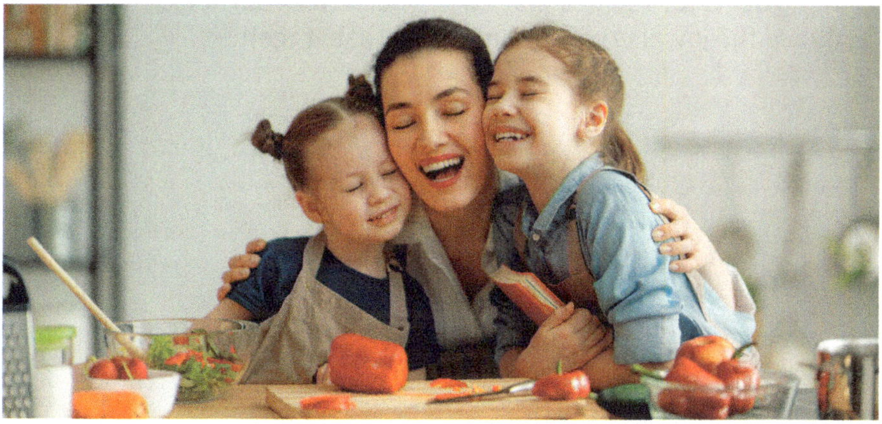

Staying Inspired

Resources and Support

Maintaining motivation can sometimes be a challenge, especially when trying to stick to a healthy eating plan. Here are a few resources to keep you inspired:

1. **Healthy Cooking Blogs:** Follow reputable health and wellness blogs that share nutritious recipes and tips for healthy living. This can provide you with new ideas and inspiration.
2. **Social Media:** Platforms like Instagram and TikTok are filled with health-conscious influencers who share their culinary adventures and creative recipes. Engage with these communities for support and inspiration.
3. **Cooking Classes:** Consider taking a cooking class focused on healthy recipes. This can be a fun way to learn new skills and meet like-minded individuals.
4. **Join a Community:** Participate in local health and wellness groups or online forums where you can share your experiences and learn from others on similar journeys.

By incorporating these tips into your routine, you can navigate social situations with confidence, involve your family in the joy of cooking, and stay inspired on your journey toward healthier eating. Let's dive into the delicious recipes that await you in this cookbook, and embrace the joy of creating nutritious treats together!

CULTURAL CONTEXT AND PERSONAL STORIES

The Role of Treats in Family Traditions

Food has a remarkable way of bringing people together, and treats often play a central role in family traditions. From birthday celebrations to holiday gatherings, desserts are often the highlight of our meals, evoking memories and creating bonds among loved ones. In my family, homemade desserts—especially frozen treats—have always been a way to celebrate special occasions and create lasting memories.

Growing up, ice cream was a staple in our household, enjoyed year-round. Whether it was a summer barbecue, a cozy winter evening, or a simple family movie night, there was always a batch of homemade ice cream ready to bring smiles to our faces. These moments fostered a sense of togetherness, where we would gather in the kitchen, share stories, and help churn the ice cream or mix in our favorite flavors. The laughter and joy shared during these times are memories I cherish and strive to recreate with my own family.

As I developed my passion for nutrition and healthy eating, I realized that I could still honor these traditions while making healthier choices. I've learned to incorporate nutritious ingredients into our beloved desserts, ensuring that we can indulge without guilt. This approach has not only allowed me to maintain family traditions but has also inspired a new generation to appreciate the joys of cooking and healthy eating.

Clara's Favorite Memories with Frozen Desserts

Among my favorite memories are the countless afternoons spent in the kitchen with my mother, experimenting with different ice cream flavors. One particular summer, we decided to create our own version of classic flavors—chocolate chip, strawberry, and mint chocolate chip. I can still recall the excitement of churning the ice cream mixture and the thrill of tasting the final product. Each flavor was a celebration of summer, and each scoop was filled with love and laughter.

Another cherished memory is the first time I introduced my daughter, Emma, to the world of homemade ice cream. I was eager to share the joy of creating something special together. We made a batch of vanilla ice cream and added her favorite mix-ins—rainbow sprinkles and cookie dough. Watching her light up with joy as she scooped her creation and shared it with the family was a heartwarming experience. It reminded me of my childhood and reinforced the importance of passing down these traditions.

These experiences have shaped my approach to nutrition and cooking. They remind me that food is more than just sustenance; it is a way to connect, celebrate, and create memories that last a lifetime. As you explore the recipes in The Nutritionist Ninja Creami Cookbook, I encourage you to create your own traditions in the kitchen, involving your family in the process of making delicious, healthy treats that will bring joy and nourishment to your lives.

ADDITIONAL RESOURCES

Recommended Healthy Cooking Blogs and Influencers

To keep your inspiration flowing, here are some of my favorite healthy cooking blogs and influencers that provide a wealth of resources, recipes, and tips for nutritious eating:

1. **minimalistbaker.com:** This blog focuses on simple, quick recipes that require 10 ingredients or less, are easily accessible, and are often plant-based. It's a fantastic resource for those looking to simplify their cooking without sacrificing flavor.
2. **ohsheglows.com:** This award-winning blog features a variety of wholesome, plant-based recipes that are both nourishing and delicious. Angela Liddon, the creator, shares personal stories and tips for healthy living that resonate with many readers.
3. **fitfoodiefinds.com:** A great source for healthy recipes that don't skimp on flavor, this blog offers a wide variety of meal ideas, meal prep tips, and fitness inspiration to help you stay on track with your health goals.
4. **nutritionstripped.com:** Run by registered dietitian McKel Kooienga, this blog focuses on whole foods and balanced nutrition. It offers a wealth of resources, including meal plans, recipes, and wellness tips that are rooted in science.

By exploring these blogs and influencers, you can find endless inspiration and support on your journey to healthier eating. They provide a sense of community, new ideas, and innovative recipes that will keep you excited about cooking and nourishing your body.

CONCLUSION

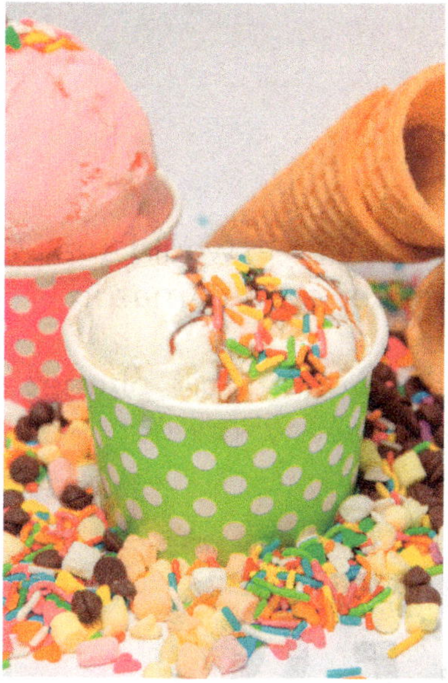

Celebrating Healthy Eating with the Ninja Creami

As we conclude this culinary journey, I hope you feel inspired to create delicious and nutritious frozen treats with your Ninja Creami. Remember, healthy eating is not about deprivation; it's about finding joy in nourishing your body with wholesome ingredients. Each recipe in this cookbook is designed to bring happiness and health to your table.

Thank You and Encouragement for Your Culinary Journey

Thank you for choosing The Nutritionist Ninja Creami Cookbook. I encourage you to continue exploring new flavors, experimenting with ingredients, and sharing your creations with family and friends. Let this book be a source of inspiration as you embrace a healthier lifestyle filled with delightful treats that nourish both body and soul.

Here's to many joyful moments spent in the kitchen, delicious treats enjoyed with family and friends, and a healthier future ahead! Happy scooping!

Hi There!

I hope you are enjoying my book so far. I would really appreciate it if you could leave a quick review on Amazon.

Just simply scan the code below using your mobile phone's camera, or you can enter the link below on our web browser.

https://swiy.com/ReviewCreami2

Thanks a lot!

- Clara

INDEX

The Index is designed to help you quickly locate specific recipes, ingredients, and topics within The Nutritionist's Ninja Creami Healthy Recipes Cookbook 2025: Healthy Guilt-Free Treats with Nutritious Ingredients. Whether you're searching for a particular frozen treat, looking for recipes that fit dietary restrictions, or exploring various ingredient options, this index will guide you efficiently to what you need.

A

B

C

D

This index is structured to help you navigate through the delightful recipes and useful information contained within this cookbook. Whether you're in search of a specific frozen treat or looking to explore new flavor combinations, simply refer to the index to find what you need quickly and easily.

Made in the USA
Monee, IL
03 November 2026

67384558R00046